SWINGING

THE GAMES YOUR NEIGHBOURS PLAY

SWINGING

THE GAMES YOUR NEIGHBOURS PLAY

MARK BRENDON

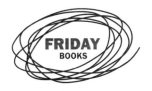

FRIDAY
BOOKS

The Friday Project
An imprint of HarperCollins Publishers
77–85 Fulham Palace Road
Hammersmith, London W6 8JB
www.thefridayproject.co.uk
www.harpercollins.co.uk

First published by The Friday Project in 2008

A catalogue record for this book is available from the British Library

ISBN 978-1-90-632113-0

Internal design and typesetting by Maggie Dana

Printed and bound in Great Britain by Clays Ltd, St Ives plc

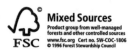

Mixed Sources
Product group from well-managed
forests and other controlled sources
www.fsc.org Cert no. SW-COC-1806
© 1996 Forest Stewardship Council
FSC

FSC is a non-profit international organisation established to promote the
responsible management of the world's forests. Products carrying the FSC
label are independently certified to assure consumers that they come from
forests that are managed to meet the social, economic and ecological
needs of present or future generations.

Find out more about HarperCollins and the environment at
www.harpercollins.co.uk/green

ABOUT THE AUTHOR

Mark Brendon is a much-travelled poet and author who has written in many genres.

He ventured tentatively into the world of swinging on leaving rehab for alcohol, and was pleasantly surprised to find it intelligent, congenial, funny, orderly, often very erotic and 'a downright sensible solution to many of the problems in a society where loneliness and frustration are institutionalised and meaningless nineteenth-century conventions still ruin many lives'.

For those readers who are still curious about this scene and would like to have a look around for themselves, I have negotiated a special free trial membership of SDC, the world's largest swingers' organisation. You may love it or hate it, but you will at least discover that the members are human.

ACKNOWLEDGEMENTS

My thanks to all who welcomed me into their homes in order to make this book possible and who, by their openness, good humour, generosity, gentleness and playfulness, made the learning process so much fun. Special thanks to Georgette Roefs, who started my instruction decades ago and has remained a loyal friend ever since, to Caroline Smailes who got the point at once and whose occasional wriggles have guided me quite as much as her astute textual criticisms, to Baz and Jayne, Chris and Theresa, Lynne at Chams – to all my delightful travelling companions and 'playmates' along the way, and, of course, to St Jude …

PART I

1

INTRODUCTION AND APOLOGIA

LAST NIGHT, MY GIRLFRIEND CHRISTY and I were having sex with a woman – mid-thirties, toned, blonde.

The blonde woman was lying on her back on a bed, hands fluttering at my hip-bones. She had slender legs encased in black hold-up stockings, a rose tattooed on her left inner thigh, a plush, shaven pussy on which we had both been lavishing attention for a good twenty minutes, a diamante ring in her belly-button, and a sweet smile.

Neither of us could actually see that smile just then, because another girl was sitting on it – one pair of lips athwart another.

This other girl was naked and tanned deep copper, with a sliver of white skin left by the tiniest of briefs. She had short, spiky, dark brown hair.

She had introduced herself to us half an hour earlier as Laurie. She had shaken our hands then, pecked our cheeks, said 'Hi! So, where are you from?'

Now she hung, gasping, her right hand gripping my left shoulder, her left on the nape of Christy's neck. Her tongue lit a tangled fuse up my throat and along my jawbone and occasionally slithered into my mouth as we both – in our different ways – used the woman beneath us for our pleasure.

The blonde woman's tongue emerged to flicker at, and to writhe into, the cleft above it, vanished then returned like a gale-blown flame.

Christy was on her hands and knees at right angles to us. Ducking down beneath Laurie, she nuzzled at the blonde woman's breasts and stomach while her left hand reached down to finger the prone woman's clitoris. She grinned up at me, then turned her head upward to kiss and nibble at Laurie's nipples.

Christy's body was being jerked and breath and sound forced from her by the man kneeling behind her. This was Laurie's boyfriend, who was – I think – called Steve. He was as fair as she was dark, with a bang of fair honey-coloured flopping over his face. He was not Christy's type, and he did what he was doing monotonously, as though he had just one gear. He said 'Yeah,' each time his belly slapped against her buttocks. That was monotonous too. She did not even look at him. She was concentrating on the feasting and the sensations up front.

Beyond us, on wall-to-wall mattresses, seven or eight naked couples were intertwined and grunting, giggling or moaning. Behind them again, against the wall, clothed couples stood watching, the men's arms hanging limply over the women's shoulders, the women occasionally moving to raise their lips like nymphing trout to kiss their men.

One woman was squatting on the carpet at my right. Her head bobbed to and fro at the groins of two men who stood upright against the wall. Her eyes, however, constantly swivelled to the scene at the centre of the room.

It was all really quite pleasant and, by most standards I think, interesting.

• • •

Christy pulled herself away from this Steve and rolled onto her back. She grinned up at me again, then pulled herself down the bed until her arse was on the very edge and her feet on the carpet. She vanished from my sight. A moment later her hair, then her nose, pushed at my testicles. Her mouth was warm and wet.

Steve had obviously followed her, because I felt her head banged rhythmically against the blonde girl's groin.

I moaned, I suppose.

A quavering male voice close at hand bleated, 'Er, darling ...?'

Christy withdrew her head from between my legs. It was cold without her there.

The man who addressed us wore a grey shirt, fawn chinos and carpet slippers. His hair was white, his face soft and pink. He fingered the gold-rimmed spectacles that hung beneath his chest.

Bending down in front of me, he crossly addressed Laurie's stomach and shaven pubis, which now slithered back and forth, a couple of feet away from his face – much closer to his wife's. 'Darling? Darling? Look, we really must be going. It's half-past one. The sitter ...'

Laurie politely raised her crotch and propped herself up on one leg so that the blonde woman could speak.

She raised her head a few inches. Her lower face gleamed. She licked her lips. 'Oh, come on, Roger,' she said. 'Give us a break. Oh, yeah ...' she creaked at me. 'No, don't stop, hun ...' Her eyes shifted back to her husband. 'I mean, fuck the sitter. I am not going 'til these guys have come.'

She pulled her right arm back through Laurie's legs, hooked it around her thigh and, with a deep laugh and an imperious 'Bring that thing back, darling ...' pulled her back down on her.

Roger took a step backward. He sighed. 'It's always the same,' he told me with a shrug and a flap. 'I mean, it's alright for you guys, but some of us have to work.'

I leaned forward on my hands. 'I know,' I panted sympathetically as my cock slid in and out of his wife. 'Still – oh, yes – you'll be able to have a lie-in tomorrow, won't you?'

'Me? Lie-in? Ha! Forget it. I've got to take Tom to cricket, then I'm meant to be driving in a road-race in Devon. And I have to be up at seven on Monday morning to get to work. And the bloody sitter charges double time after midnight.'

My lips were working as I tried to stop myself from laughing.

This was swinging for you. Middle-class concerns with children and domestic budgets in amongst the groans and yelps of orgiasts.

'Yes,' I said sympathetically. 'Wish I could get that sort of money for sitting on my arse ... doing ... mmm ... nothing ...'

Roger nodded. He had found a friend. 'Well, do be as quick as you can, will you?' he said. 'If she lets you ...'

I nodded obediently.

Roger shuffled away towards the door. 'Oh, and Karen!' he turned and raised his voice. He spoke very slowly, as though to a very old foreigner. 'I've got your bag, OK? And your shoes are outside the dark room.' He shook his head sorrowfully, and told me, 'She's always losing things ...'

As he shuffled from the room, Christy allowed a giggle to bubble up. She knelt up at my shoulder so that I felt her pussy damp and hot against my buttocks. Her fingers plucked at my nipples. 'Come on, darling,' she croaked in my ear. 'For heaven's sake, think about the sitter ...'

Laurie's hand reached out for mine and clasped it. She grit her teeth. Beneath her, Karen said, 'Hmmff,' and burbled. Christy and I laughed and kissed. Laurie leaned forward. Her tongue joined ours and slithered around them. Her eyes sparkled, so I kissed them too.

Group hug, only naked and interlinked by tongues and genitals. We were all four united in playful naughtiness and companionship. In that moment, surely, we loved one another.

2

TAMING LUST

TO DATE ALMOST ALL the books and articles about swinging have been written by panting 'vanillas' (as non-swingers are known) alternately – or sometimes simultaneously – drooling and expressing disapproval.

Theirs is surely the most disreputable form of journalism. Peeking in, urging on those observed, picking out the saleable or sensational aspects of its subjects' activities, then retreating to don an enemy padre's uniform.

This book's purpose is not to titillate – or, at least, not directly. If it opens up new prospects and inspires individuals or couples to conjure their own fantasies and make their own plans for sexual adventure, I am delighted. But it features few detailed accounts of sex, and studiously avoids the lyrical when it does so.

I include the mundane little memoir of last night because, commonplace though it is, it summarises much of what swinging is about. There is the sensuality, of course, and the curiosity as to the sexuality of others. There are the senses of adventure and community and, perhaps above all, the affectionate playfulness ...

It also typifies the essential conventionality of swingers.

Swingers by definition respect the sanctity – or, at least, the value – of secure, enduring marriage or partnership, and the requirements of children. They do not have extra-marital affairs, nor allow their emotions to be influenced by their sexual needs by falling 'in love' with their secretaries, gardeners, colleagues, personal trainers, spouse's best friends or children's schoolfellows, to the peril of their homes and their children's welfare.

They recognise, however, that the extended family has gone, the nuclear family couple is insufficient to meet their emotional and sexual needs, and the active sex-life-expectancy has been enormously prolonged over the past two centuries. For those reasons they cannot find all the adventure, interest and passion they require in one person, who inevitably has distinct needs and develops at a different pace from themselves.

They therefore seek mutuality in shared sexual adventures.

Let's face it: it is a lot more amusing, convivial and revealing than, say, golf or fishing. And, while these have in large measure been gender-specific distractions – or refuges – from hearth and home, swinging is by definition a cross-gender and wholly mutual diversion.

It takes lust – the wolf that snuffles and growls at the door of every marital home – tames it, and brings it into the house as an amusing and stimulating pet.

To the seeker of pornography, those four or five bodies intertwined on the bed last night were merely performing an undifferentiated thing called sex. For those bodies' owners, however, it was a celebration of one another, of the infinite variety of human responses and sensuous experience, and of their own strength, vivacity and beauty within that fleeting moment.

And it was without recrimination or cost – except for babysitting fees.

It was loving, laughing and irresponsible.

It was play.

3

IT IS EVERYWHERE

SHOW ME AN URBAN TERRACE, suburban close or sleepy village, and I will show you swingers. In every city, market-town and village in the Western world and beyond, there are respectable groups, couples and singles who routinely engage in recreational sex with total strangers, or with people encountered for that purpose just minutes before.

In time many of them become friends and, like any other social group, hold little parties at which they frequently run into one another, or invite one another over as if for supper. So Derek and Joan will ring Tony and Sharon and suggest that they come over for a drink and maybe a little shag.

'Oh, and there's this rather nice new couple who've just moved into the area ... Nothing fancy. Just the six of us. And we can't go on too late because Joan has to be in Westminster by eleven tomorrow ...'

Sometimes these couples will go on holiday together, and perhaps they will go out one night to a Spanish, Mexican or Dominican swing-club to whoop it up with the locals. Sometimes they will go to Cap d'Agde – the French town wholly dedicated to nudism and swinging – or to one of many resorts and hotels throughout the world providing for 'the Lifestyle' ...

There are millions of swingers worldwide (four million is the generally accepted estimate in the US alone) and many millions more who are curious about the lifestyle, or aspire to become part of it. It has become perhaps the Western world's biggest and most rapidly booming subculture – and its most widespread secret.

Although they are to be counted only in their thousands, ferret-keepers and Civil War enthusiasts, steam-train afficianados and cryptographers seeking to unravel the Beale code all have their own publications. For many reasons, however, there are few – if any – books by a practising swinger offering bona fide, sympathetic information and an insight into this massive social phenomenon.

The problem is that swingers are, by nature and long habit, discreet.

They may be unashamed – even proud – of their activities and of their fellows. They may know that the law protects them from overt discrimination. They, like 'homosexual' men and women, are adults engaged in an entirely consensual leisure activity which is – or, at least, should be – nobody's business but their own.

So, of course, were foxhunters and bareheaded motorcyclists, but that didn't prevent government and illiberal moralists from pretending that it was the welfare of the fox or the rider that warranted their intervention (though they have shown no such concern for battery hens).

Swingers have no prey. Even the commonplace transaction with a prostitute, the making of pornography, the habitual wine-bar or clubbing seduction, may be exploitative of one who, by reason of age, idiocy, poverty, drug-addiction, emotional need or *force majeure*, is in fact unwilling or reluctant. Swingers, however, play exclusively with other adults who have chosen this lifestyle. They obtain explicit consent before any sexual contact.

Yet for all this, most swingers are unwilling to subject themselves or their families to the censorious and lubricious judgements of the media who, at one level, cringe like adolescents from acknowledgement of genitals (unless they are swathed in white slipper satin for religious ceremony or shaven and sanctified by 'the miracle of birth'), and at the other, gawp at them with yearning but profess outrage at their functions.

Sex may be the throbbing heart of our marketing and media culture, invariably – and oh, how wrongly – presented as desirable. We may regularly expose poor, bare, forked man – and woman – but, when we come to acknowledging that we actually have sexual functions and emissions, we might as well still be dressed as china bells.

Over the past three years, while researching for this book, I have been a swinger. In the course of this period, I have visited many private parties and most of Britain's principal swingers' clubs, as well as hotels, beaches and resorts throughout Britain and beyond where adults openly engage in sexual play.

I have had sex (in Clintonian and non-Clintonian senses) or – as swingers have it – I have 'played' with several hundreds of female strangers and acquaintances with whom I have little or no other connection. Sometimes they have been alone, sometimes in pairs. Sometimes there have been as many as seven or eight in one afternoon or evening. Quite often, I have known their forenames before I did so.

I have generally done so in the presence of my girlfriend and these women's husbands or boyfriends. And at the orgies that are our principal diversions, we have been amidst forty, fifty or sixty or more couples, most of them naked or sparsely clothed, and similarly engaged.

Tabloid journalists pruriently 'investigating' the swing-scene always 'make their excuses and leave'. I have stayed. I make no excuses for it. It has been instructive, companionable and often great fun.

I could pretend to dispassion or disdain. I could now clamber back onto the raft of respectability and express disapproval of the swinging lifestyle. This would be both dishonest and unconvincing.

Yes, sometimes the experience has been banal, squalid and depressing, but the same could be said of regular eating out or concert-going. This has been a function of peculiar people or circumstances, not of the activity itself.

In general, I have found swingers amiable. They are sensualists and libertarians, unembarrassed and intent on sharing pleasures with childlike openness. Given its ubiquity and the diversity of its practitioners, however, swinging inevitably has its share of crass berks and power-hungry bitches who believe that tantra is a plural.

But only in societies where responsibility has been usurped by law can such people thrive. Subcultures, if not illegal, are without the law. Swinging is therefore dependent on reciprocity and is self-policing. In my experience, such people are soon ostracised and find themselves on the grimy fringes of the movement. Should you find yourself amongst them, simply leave. Their faults are not those of the milieu which, in general, I have found to be good-natured and enormous fun.

4

AFFECTION, FLIRTATION, ADVENTURE ...

I WAS 47 YEARS OLD when I set out on this journey. I had been married for seven miserable years and divorced for twelve, ten of which I had spent in a more or less monogamous relationship. Now, on leaving rehab for alcohol dependence, I was alone.

• • •

'Sex is just another quick fix ...' my counsellor told me on my last morning at the clinic.

Emma was charming, sympathetic, proficient, almost prim. I had to remind myself that before she became sober, she had lived the usual junky life of blurry jags, blags and shags on the streets. Now she crossed stockinged legs beneath her desk and wiggled the lavalliere at her throat.

'... just another quick fix, another way of refusing to look at yourself and who you really are. As you know, it can be an addiction too.'

I shook my head. It was during my three-month stay in the clinic that my long-term girlfriend at last decided – really quite reasonably – that she had had enough. I was confronting a solitary existence out there.

'Cocteau used to complain that he was asked to travel on a filthy, cramped train to nowhere,' I told Emma, 'but when he took opium, he was enabled to jump off and sit on the banks amidst the flowers, yet here were all these people urging him to get back on the train. I understand why it is not a good idea to take opium or alcohol if you are an addict, but I don't understand why it is invariably bad to get off, stretch your legs and breathe the fresh air.'

'Sex can be just as dangerous as alcohol or opium,' she said.

'I'm sure it can, Em, but so can food or oxygen in excess. Doesn't alter the fact that they are also essentials. And sex is – or it can be – a very good thing. It's a loving thing, an adventure, a great game when played between equals and friends, a madness in controlled circumstances. It lets you escape from the paltry, transitory concerns and the isolation of every day. I think I can now live without alcohol, but I really don't think that I can live without sex. You've just levelled all the mountains in my landscape. Now you seem to be telling me that I should cut down the trees as well. Just a featureless desert ...'

'No, no, no,' she soothed. 'We're not saying that you must avoid sex. Just relationships – and just for the time being.'

Outside on the gravel drive my fellow-patients sloped out of the front door and slumped onto benches or sprawled on the sun-dappled lawns to smoke and shake and chat.

'Look, I know the rules,' I said, 'but I don't understand them. No "relationships" for at least twelve months, and then only with a pot-plant. Then an undemanding pet like a hamster, then a dog, and finally another human being ... And you say we don't have to avoid sex? That pot-plant had better be a cactus.'

Emma intoned it like a catechism response. 'Sex for its own sake is just using another person to escape from reality ...'

'Yes? And? Flying is just an escape from the equally inexorable forces of gravity. It can take you somewhere you want to go, or you can just go for a whirl, land where you took off, and it gives you a thrill and a beautiful view of the world. And if it's mutual?'

'... and you need to focus on who you are, what you need for happiness, and that must come from inside you. You need to find peace and serenity within yourself.'

'Certainly, but myself is a sexual being. Serene isn't exactly easy when you're shaking with longing every time you see a frolicsome sheep.'

'Hey, no! I'm not expecting you to be totally celibate ...'

'Thank you.'

'... but only on the strict condition that you don't give the other person power over your contentment or emotional stability. Your life depends upon that.'

'I know that. I realise that,' I nodded. 'But listen, Em. I still want to share large aspects of my life. I want affection and adventure and flirtation. I want freedom. Are you saying I should just be a brutal, uncaring exploiter, then? Hurting others who expect more of me? Love 'em and leave 'em, and to hell with the consequences? Is that how you ensure the next generation of patients here?'

'No, of course not,' she smiled indulgently.

'So, sex but no relationships? Which means – what? Whores?'

'No!' She reconsidered. She gulped. 'Well, maybe. Possibly. But that can leave you feeling lonely and degraded. Just someone strong and not needy ...'

'I turn gay, then?'

'That's not fair.' Her lips writhed. She did unnecessary things with papers and smiled. 'Look, Mark, there are many people of both genders who can give love without sex and can share sex without regarding it as proof of ownership or allowing it to become a replacement obsession. It shouldn't be such a big deal for you ... You must never allow it to take the place of your Higher Power.'

'Frustrated desire is far more likely to do that,' I told her. 'Not desire for sex, as such, but desire for the warmth, the closeness, the laughter, the excitement ...'

'Precisely,' she said, as if it meant or proved anything. 'The excitement ...' She leaned across the desk and laid a hand on my forearm. 'It's all right,' she added, 'you'll work it out.'

5

'NONE OF US WANTED OWNERSHIP ...'

TWO MONTHS LATER, I was living sober and alone in a Somerset country cottage with a greyhound and sixteen laying hens. I was still no closer to working it out.

I shared my counsellor's views on dependent, grasping, vampiric relationships. I did not want to feign love or, ever again, to feel that my happiness depended entirely upon that of another human being, or vice versa.

But neither did I want casual sex with strangers or – still worse – friends, and the resultant feelings of waste and emptiness.

I had tried it, of course, since I had been sober. It is not hard today to find another pair of eyes in which needs – for validation, for comfort, for adventure, for belief – glimmer as they circle just beneath the bright surface sparkle.

Six such pairs of eyes, then, had gazed up at mine from my groin and had rolled upward into momentary unconsciousness as their owners knelt or splayed like starfish beneath me.

Two of these women had husbands, which was ideal, but one of them was already talking about leaving her husband – not to move in with me, of course. That would be far too gauche for a modern girl. No, but flats in town were hard to find. Maybe she could find somewhere just down the road from me ...

As for the remainder, two had left earrings on the first night, one her 'special' knickers. This merely demonstrated touching fidelity to convention.

I too had never wanted one-night stands, nor regarded sex as so rare as to be desirable in itself. We were all agreed, then. But in that case, given that we wanted neither casual sex nor exclusivity and dependence, just what did we want?

Well, I wanted to give each of them a key to my house so that she could turn up when she felt like it, sit and read or listen to music, slip into bed beside me when she wanted a chat, a cuddle or a fuck. I wanted a best friend who loved every part of me.

I liked it when they cleaned my kitchen or changed the bed-linen in my absence. I loved it when they made friends with my dog. Did each such intimacy mean that I must further cut myself off from them because I was forced to deceive? What if two of them turned up on the same night? Must I then scamper around like the asinine husband of French farce, keeping them apart and hiding evidence? Must I conceal from each a large part of my nature and my life?

And they too did not want – well, maybe the jewellery shop manageress who gradually colonised my drawers with her clothes did, but more by reflex than reason – to live happily ever after with me and to bear my children. They did not want me questioning them as to where they had been and what they had done with whom.

None of us wanted ownership, but we all valued affection and courtesy and did not want to cause hurt. On the other hand, we were all sexually active and desirous and had – whatever this may mean – a great need to give and to share love. We craved adventure. We needed to explore other human territories. We wanted the freedom, the sanction, the blessing afforded by the acceptance of ourselves naked, unguarded, needy and wild.

I would never marry again. I was pretty sure of that. I doubted, even, that I would ever live with anyone in the long term. I would spend a great deal of my life alone. Once I could cope with the reflex temptations to drink, I would no doubt venture down to the pub to sit sober and hope to fascinate or meet people through my work, and form transitory attachments.

At times, she – whoever she might be – would become more dependent and demanding than I could stand, and the relationship would founder amidst grief and recriminations. At times, through weakness or chivalry, I would encourage such dependence, only to check myself and arduously to unravel the knots that I had so laboriously tied.

There would, I supposed, be occasional prostitutes. This, too, would be a moral choice. I would opt for any halfway house which would acknowledge my nature yet obviate needless damage to myself or to others.

It was not an exciting prospect, but it was all that I could allow myself.

But at that point – one grey, rain-spangled morning – the gods took a kindly hand.

6

A WHORE AND A VAGABOND

LISA WAS 36 AT THE TIME.

She was a whore and a vagabond.

She was also, amongst other things, an occasional psychiatric nurse, a registered childminder and a very good guitarist. She lived for the most part in a bright yellow Bedford van.

She was part Romany on her mother's side, gorgio on her father's, with a sizeable slug of Afro-Caribbean in the mix. This made her hair black, lustrous and curly and her skin the colour of wet sand and silkier than any other I have ever encountered.

Her father was a non-conformist minister, a Biblical scholar, a *Grateful Dead*-head and a former hippy with teeth like sunset Dolomites. I had met him at a lecture tht I had given in Manchester. He approached me afterwards to correct my interpretation of a text in Acts and to explain some hitherto unsuspected meanings – probably unsuspected even by Jerry Garcia – in *Dark Star*. For a grizzled, bearded minister of God, he could certainly down the Bushmills and played a mean game of pool.

At the time, during my year's separation from my long-term girl-friend before I went into rehab, I was living near Bath. Somewhere in the evening Gordon Shavalar had leaned on my shoulder and told me, through hot fluffy breath, that I should look up his daughter who was mostly based down west these days.

I had taken him at his word.

Lisa and I had met six or seven months before I had enrolled at the clinic. We had at once been attracted.

She was a laconic, luxuriant sort of girl with a slender, athletic but sensuous frame, ornate tattoos on her left shoulder and down her right upper arm, forearms taut and sinewy as a hare's, and a funny little rag doll face which suddenly sprang into life with a happy smile or a mock-sardonic sneer.

Clothes looked uncomfortable and ungainly on her. Remove them, and she moved with an imperious degree of self-possession and a childlike natural elegance. She did not draw in her little round stomach or extend a hand to protect herself as she shambled about naked or in bra and knickers. She clothed herself in nudity. She wore it beautifully. She was a very lovely animal to watch.

And she was a lovely animal with whom to make love – for that, mysteriously, was what we had found ourselves doing.

I don't know how it happens, how first the caressing and kissing and fucking move into synch, so that ferocity and tenderness, hunger and savour, adult and child, human and beast, male and female all coexist and intermingle. Then suddenly, fear and need and all the horrors and vulnerability are also offered up for inspection and approval, are blessed, sanctioned and loved, and memories from before birth – and maybe from before language – emerge, are recognised and find their echoes. Then distinctions vanish and you gaze into her eyes, and something deep within her says 'Yes' and opens up to babies or to death, or to whatever acceptance may bring, and you are lost and home, all at once.

Which is a crappy mess of an explanation, but, if I could express it any better, it would not be worth doing. And, oh, it was. It is.

'God,' she had said, 'I really like that energy.' I did not understand this, but since other women have said much the same thing and since the energy is mine, I accepted it without objection.

And so she had stayed, sometimes for as long as four whole days. Then she would start to be brisk and dismissive as she created distance between us so that she could escape, because her independence and her solitude were more sacred to her than anything else.

And for weeks after her departure, if I called her on her mobile, it was, 'Yes. What was it?' and I would find myself cut off if I so much as dared to try to chat companionably. On one occasion, she reiterated without the least prompting, 'It's not as if we made love or anything. I mean, yes, it's good sex, but for fuck's sake, man ...'

Sometimes she just fled so that she could be back in her wagon, with its little wood-burning stove and its bookcase with ropes anchoring each rank of books, and its tutus and flowery frocks hanging from the ceiling, and whips and giant patent fetish-boots tucked away beneath the bed.

She would spend whole weeks just parked in a copse somewhere, smoking dope and chilling and 'being real'.

Sometimes she headed off with fellow-travellers to find a location for a rave or 'free party' out in the country and to send out the secret mobile phone messages that draw 'cheesy quavers' in from all over the country. I went to one of these with her – just two days and nights of drifting and dancing and sleeping, rough feasting and occasional, incidental fucking in the woods, all to the sounds of trance and techno and drum'n'bass. I liked everything except the sounds.

Sometimes – for two or three months at a time, and for two or three days a week – she would take a job as a 'working girl' in a massage parlour.

'Yeah, I'm proud of giving good value,' she told me. 'I can disconnect so it doesn't touch me, but that doesn't mean I don't give them what they need.'

Once I introduced her to a dear old friend, a paediatric sister at Great Ormond Street Hospital for Children. The two women got on well. They teased me relentlessly. They walked the dog a lot together. Tilly, my nurse friend, came to a conclusion that surprised her. 'I don't know if it's genetic, or a product of upbringing and experience,' she said, 'a deficiency or an attribute, but she and I are the same. Loads of women say to me about my job, "How can you give so much to a dying child, then come in and find him gone and his bed occupied by another, and just keep on giving?" So I get accused of being heartless and unnatural in the same breath as I'm called an angel and a saint.

'And Lisa does the same, and she's accused of being unnatural too. She's a carer and gets paid for it. She just has that ability – like me – to cut herself off in order to survive. It doesn't make her any less sincere or valuable, and she gets called all sorts of unpleasant names too.

'It's a female thing, I think. I don't know. Maybe that's just conditioning, but the caring thing is always associated with females and so is the ability to disconnect. So in some of us, the two exist side by side. Maybe we're more highly developed than other women. Maybe we're less developed – throwbacks or something. Either way, I reckon the world should be bloody glad we exist ...'

Lisa had always told me (like a cross between Mary Poppins and Aslan, which is quite appropriate really), 'One day, I'll just be gone.'

One day, six weeks before I went to the clinic, she was. Her mobile number was unobtainable.

So what did I do? I, of course, got drunk, and damned her.

• • •

But that clogged Mancunian voice awoke me at ten o'clock that gloomy, sober morning. 'Hi, baby boy! How's it going? You off the sauce now, darlin'? How was the Gulag, then?'

'Lisa,' I croaked, then sat up and cleared my throat. Rainwater was chuckling as it streamed from the gutter outside my window. 'God, Lisa! How ...? Hey, how are you?'

'I'm OK. Saw your mate Tim in Ashburton the other day. He told me where you were ...'

'You just evaporated last time,' I said. 'I thought you'd gone for good.'

'Always told you, didn't I? I come and go ...'

'Oh, come, darling, come! Where'd you get to? Where are you now?'

'Could be with you in an hour, actually,' she said. 'Be really nice to see you ... Yeah, go on. Shitty day. Give me directions and get the coffee pot on ...'

I whooped as I laid down the receiver.

• • •

It took Lisa just half an hour to have the fire lit in the sitting-room and to be in her usual state of undress in a red lacy bra and knickers.

If there was contrivance or sexual intent there, it was carried lightly. She knew that I enjoyed watching her. She enjoyed being watched and the sensations and the freedom of nakedness.

She lay open, her limbs petals to a flower in full bloom. Her head and shoulders were raised on brocade cushions. One knee was raised, the other hooked and sagging off the sofa. Her left hand lolled at the scarlet, lacy escarpment at her groin. Her right held a joint on which she drew deep.

She had looked around the house and pronounced it 'OK'. She had become quite excited about the still intact water-heating copper in the pantry. She had been in Avignon, she said, for the Festival, and had then wandered on down into Italy, but had not yet been ready to set off on her long discussed 'big trip' to Romania (where she hoped to buy a patch of land), and on through the Russias.

She had returned just two weeks earlier, and had already found a massage parlour in Taunton where she now worked for a couple of days a week. She was also busy organising a huge late-summer rave, somewhere in the Wiltshire downs.

I sat at my desk, telling her of the struggles of rehab and responding to – or, more often, deleting – emails. Concentration was not easy with those gaping thighs, inexorably framing and leading the eye to their apex.

I swivelled my chair round. 'Just what is it,' I asked her in admittedly fatuous frustration, 'about pussy?'

She giggled and shrugged. 'Well, if you don't know, I don't reckon I can tell you.'

'No, I know it's a daft question, but really, where does the visual power come from? Striptease, the can-can, the fan-dance, the split skirt, the miniskirt, they all posit a desire to see this somehow climactic organ. Men and women alike, we all crane and strain for that moment of revelation, but of what?'

'Nuts, isn't it?'

'Very specifically, no.'

'Tee hee. S'pose not.'

'Anyhow, your arrival is a boon and blessing,' I told her. 'Not just because I love to see you, but because, for once, you're not forbidden fruit. If women were available on prescription, I'd be told to take two of you before meals ...'

'Hey. Not sure I like that,' she said ruefully. 'I like to be forbidden, or, at least, exotic ...'

'Oh, darling, you are all of that,' I growled.

'... not sort of standard issue therapeutic. You mean this not being allowed to have a relationship bit? Well, yeah, at least you know that I'm not going to want to move in or depend on you or anyone else.'

'Exactly. Straight out of the text-books. Ex-addict's dream ...'

'You should be an escort in the States,' she said suddenly. 'My mate Annabel said that a while back when she heard your voice on the phone. She's right, too. That voice, that energy, you'd make a fortune ...'

'You reckon?' I considered the irresponsible vision that her words conjured. 'I'd almost do that, you know, if it didn't just mean fat, blue-rinsed matrons, endless Viagra and the slow death of the soul. Lots of sex, adventure, lots of new, interesting people ...'

'Yeah, you're good at the giving bit,' she said dreamily, readjusting the cushions so that she could lie back, 'just no good at having things taken from you. Good at the excitement and the novelty, bad at the day-to-day grind ...'

And that is when she said it.

She said, 'You ought to try swinging, you know. Probably not standard therapy, but you'd like it ...'

'I don't know ...' I frowned, but yes, my heartbeat quickened.

On the one hand, the word evoked associations with freedom, sensuality and uncritical acceptance. I had enjoyed just eight very happy threesomes to date, and I had loved the experiences. There had been no pleading or striving for acceptance or pardon. Sexuality had simply been acknowledged, shared and celebrated.

On the other hand, I associated the organised version with shame-faced suburban desperation, sleaze and squalor.

I said, 'It always sounded like fun in theory ...'

'So, why not?'

'Ah, I wouldn't know where to start,' I said, very much hoping that she might have a few suggestions, 'and I'm too ancient, aren't I?'

'Of course you're not! Fuck, there are swingers out there well into their sixties. You'd be a breath of fresh air. Decent looks, manners, slim. Answer to a maiden's prayer, you.'

'Yeah, yeah. Well, I would like to try ...' I sidestepped out from behind the desk. I picked up my mug. As I bent to lift hers from the coffee-table, I kissed the top of her head. She raised her lips to kiss mine with a 'Mmmmm'.

'Anyhow,' I asked, as I headed for the kitchen. 'How do you know all this? Swinging's not your scene, is it?'

She cocked her head this way and that. 'Er, yes and no,' she replied. 'I mean, it's a counter-culture, isn't it? And there are real people on that scene. And they're seekers, aren't they? And the sex – the erotic stuff, the sights and stuff – can be really good.'

I walked into the kitchen, leaving the door open behind me. I flicked on the kettle and rinsed the mugs under the tap. 'But yeah,' she called over the sofa-back and her arm, 'it's mostly sort of middle-class and can be scared and up its own arse. But, you know, we're talking people trying to face their fears and be what they are. I prefer the free party scene. Less accent on the sex there. Sex is just, you know, one of the means of expression, and everyone is just mad. The swing-scene, it's like "We're all mad and free but in a sane and respectable way", you know?'

'But how – when were you involved?'

'Oh, shit. You can't not be. You point me at ten houses, I'll find you at least one swinging couple.'

I made the coffee and headed back into the sitting-room. 'So, would you give me a hand?' I asked casually. 'Getting started, I mean.'

She shrugged. 'Yeah, OK. You set it all up. I'm saving for a big trip, so I'm going to be around for the next six months or so. I'll do a few parties and meets with you. Give me enough notice, I'll come with you. You'll make friends quickly, though.'

And that was that.

In volunteering to escort me, Lisa was presumably volunteering to have sex with a number of males and females as yet unknown to us. This struck me as, at once, strange, shocking and exciting. I felt grateful to her. I still, for some reason, regarded such an undertaking as a sacrifice. She disabused me of the notion with a shrug. 'Sex is a pleasure, and I don't fuck people if I don't fancy them, so it's no big deal.'

No big deal to her, perhaps, but the notion that I could enjoy a full, exciting and adventurous social and sexual life, do no damage and return to privacy, hard work and freedom was enthralling.

Lisa and I went to bed at around three o'clock. Darkness fell, lives began and ended, hours and half-hours pealed about the world. We did not notice. We took breaks for cigarettes and chat, and even once to take the dog out, lock up the hens and fry a few eggs for ourselves before returning to the chaotic and cluttered bedroom to resume our joyous conversation until early morning.

I had been terrified when first I emerged from the clinic. For thirty years I had not fucked a girl without at least a glass of champagne to enhance her glamour and quiet my critical faculties. I had feared that the whole business might prove comical or simply depressing. I need not have worried. Sex was far better and more interesting and intense than in my drinking days.

And now I had the chance to join the secret, underground society of swingers.

PART II

1

SWINGING AND MORALITY

I WAS INTERESTED ... Oh, bollocks. I was fascinated and excited at the prospect.

For all my eagerness, I was properly cautious.

My experiences of addictive activities had been good, which is to say in the long term, bloody awful.

I took up smoking at fifteen in the music-school practice rooms. Now I accounted for an ounce of roll-up shag a day. I started drinking alcohol at seventeen and soon found myself downing a litre and a half of whisky, with Guinness on the side, every night. Cocaine had never been a threat. It had simply permitted greater alcohol consumption with more sex. It had just been a sauce to the principal ingredient.

Swinging seemed to me logically and emotionally desirable, but I knew that many people thought it morally reprehensible. Until now, I had never really considered why.

I discounted at once all objections from the huge majority. All those of both sexes who read or watch pornography – and they are to be counted in their billions – those who read with prurient delight of 'three-in-a-bed romps' in their newspapers, use prostitutes for sexual gratification, or regularly have sex for no better reason than hunger for sensual pleasure and shared warmth in a cold and hostile world – they all do, or dream of doing, the same things as the swing-set. It seemed to me that they should not add hypocrisy to pusillanimity.

The commonest objection raised by the remainder was that sex is, or rather should be, an exclusive and sacred activity. 'It's the highest and deepest form of communication that we've got,' wrote my old university friend, Juliette. 'With someone you love, it can be glorious. With someone else, it can be squalid and degrading.'

I put this to Lisa. 'Yeah, but is this some sort of philosophy or just a profession of psychosis?' she demanded. 'Sure, sex is better when you feel stimulated, and for lots of people that means when you feel secure. So doing it with someone you trust not to laugh at your bits, or your whimpering, nor take advantage of your vulnerability, makes it easier to let go and do it properly. So what?

'That's just like saying, back in the days when people were always poisoning one another or falling on one another in their cups, "The only good meal is one enjoyed in the bosom of your family". But that's just a reflection of fear in the world outside, not of the nature of food or eating out.'

For all that, this is the only objection to swinging to which I have had to defer.

For myself, I have known both wonderful and deeply disappointing sexual experiences with strangers, kindred spirits and enemies, but maybe others really do enjoy a transcendent experience beyond my ken. I certainly cannot disprove it, but then neither could they prove their assertion – though many act as if it were a given, like those people who have visited just one foreign country and forever afterwards insist that it is the best and that they know 'abroad'.

Sex obviously did not evolve as a means to spiritual revelation or lifetime bonding, but it can undoubtedly play a part in both. But then, the same can be said of religion. The insistence that these are the sole purposes of both, however, has given rise to ordinances that they should be performed only in certain ways and with chosen people.

And these have played a far greater role in the subjugation of genders, classes and individuals, than in that of increasing human happiness.

The commonest distinction made is that between 'making love' and fucking. The former is supposedly desirable and morally praiseworthy (the word 'love' sanctifies, though emotions claiming that name have done infinitely more damage than, say, liking), the latter reprehensible.

In fact, the distinction is simply that between good sex and bad. Good, responsive lovers make love even when they are strangers. We are human, after all – naked, needy, greedy, open and vulnerable. What in the name of God is not to love?

2

THE YUCKINESS FACTOR

I SOUGHT MORE TELLING reasons for disapproval.

The next objection I encountered was the argument from personal distaste which, of course, is not an argument at all.

'It's just – I don't know,' said my neighbour, Tess. 'It's yucky. I mean, sex just is yucky really, unless you love the person ...'

This confusion of ethical and aesthetic is common in our Disney-fied age, in which we strive to spare ourselves certain sights whose consequences we desire. And the blonde one is always the victim.

We want meat, but are outraged at the sight of death, so our animals (rather like our aged relatives) are simply locked away from our view – and that of the sun. They are tortured throughout their lives so that we should not be exposed to the momentary discomfort of witnessing their merciful deaths. Once dead, they are moulded into breadcrumbed gobbets so that our children should not be traumatised by the thought of real animals dying to feed them.

This same immoral conflation of the 'yucky' and the evil has been used to condemn abortion, homosexuality, miscegenation and even the culling of vermin. The middle-class majority finds it distasteful, therefore it is wrong.

I was reared – as were most of the current swing-set – in an age of sexual caution and obscurantism in which 'homosexuality' was criminal and scorned, females must keep their legs clamped together for fear of revealing the very fact of genitalia, and fear of pregnancy and residual notions of propriety and property dominated heterosexual dealings.

All our first sexual impulses were guided towards phallocentricity. Sex had one defining *sine qua non* – male ejaculation within just one female orifice. The notion that this orifice and related organs were in fact autonomous, with their own functions and feelings, was heresy. The availability of oral contraception was insufficient to banish the associations of pollution, pregnancy and possession.

We adolesced into an age of licence, in which sex was recognised as a pleasure, not – or not necessarily – as a sacrament.

There was a further major shift with the advent of AIDS.

I had not used a condom until well after my thirty-fifth year. They are now standard prerequisites of all penetrative sex, save within exclusive relationships, at all levels of society. The pollutant, territory-marking aspects of sex have gone, rendering oral sex often more intimate and exclusive than genital or anal.

Sex has not so much been demoted as democratised. A king may romp with children and still rule in pomp. Bouncy pop pap does not render a Bach chorale any the less sacred or moving. So, sex as a leisure activity need not devalue its own currency.

This is not to say that – as with any other pleasure – that there is no risk of its becoming a fetish or an obsession, nor that it can or should be enjoyed without regard to those with whom it is shared. Merely that, when all courtesies have been considered, it can be enjoyed rather than denied due to jealousies or artificial and, in this age, apparently meaningless conventions.

So much is now widely accepted – and, interestingly, more generally accepted it seems – by women who are empowered and independent. But they find themselves denied adequate sexual gratification, adventure or community, and increasingly resort to 'smart-casual' (within an inherently transient but orderly relationship, rather than casual or within a formal bond) sexual adventure.

Personal tastes, of course, vary widely. Some find their own bodies and those of others repugnant and consider their functions – sex no less than defecation – somehow squalid and shameful.

There may be a thousand sad reasons for such deviant idealism, but there is no reason for considering it a valid criticism. Again it tells us more of the afflicted person than of the activities despised. Sex, defecation and death exist. An aesthetic that finds them ugly, is therefore founded upon false premises. It is fantastic. It is alienated. It is neurotic. It is, in religious terms, blasphemous.

Still less arguable are the requirements of individual sexuality. Many – the porn-watchers amongst them – love to be surrounded by visual and auditory stimuli, and enjoy mild exhibitionism and voyeurism as fillips to their desire. Others prefer the security of the familiar and of privacy.

Such particularity is no more valid grounds for disapproval than a preference for meat over fish, or for one gender over another. Privacy, after all, is a very new commodity in human society – a modern (fetishistic because peripheral to the sexual act itself) requirement.

When Lisa and I questioned Tess, she conceded that her assessments of 'yuckiness' and desirability varied from circumstance to circumstance, day to day, and even hour to hour. 'I mean, I generally think eating pussy is yucky, but there've been moments ... But that's just desire blinding me, isn't it?'

She was gracious enough to admit that, for all she knew, her vision might be obscured by fear and considerations of propriety and cleared by sexual desire. Hardly the basis, then, for a constraint that could possibly be classified as 'ethical'.

3

DOES GASTRONOMY 'DEVALUE' HOME COOKING?

AT DINNER IN THEIR KITCHEN a couple of days later, Fiona – the ageless, very beautiful, Sloaney wife of a doctor friend – raised the argument that swinging somehow 'devalues' sex or the human body.

Her husband Johnny (tactfully) and I (less so) confessed that we found this one incomprehensible.

Grant that we all have sexual urges and that these are not of their nature specific. In what sense then can it be claimed that routine fulfilment of these urges within marriage or long-term relationships places a higher value on sex than what is, after all, a carefully prepared, long-anticipated, mutually exciting celebration of physical pleasures?

Johnny chose much the same metaphor as Lisa. As well argue, he said, that a celebratory dinner at a fine restaurant with food prepared by strangers 'devalues' that prepared at home by spouses.

Unsurprisingly for a doctor, Johnny placed little added value on the human body's functions. 'Look, Fi, I'm not denying there's something lovely and consoling – sacramental, if you like – about good old cottage-pie on Monday and chicken *fricassée* on Tuesday, even if the cottage-pie is watery and lumpy and the chicken bland – not that yours ever is, of course, darling. But you really can't accuse Gordon Ramsay of destroying people's pleasure in home cooking by giving them the occasional joys of exciting smells, textures and flavours in a luxurious and theatrical environment.

'So yep, OK. I actually am basically a cottage-pie man. I like all that familiarity and prolonged proximity. It's sort of the grout securing the tesserae of a relationship ...'

'But it's not to denigrate the importance of grout,' I said, 'to acknowledge that it can often be just a little dull.'

'Thank you, Mark,' said Fi. The corner of her lips twitched.

'No, come on! I'm sure you make brilliant steak and kidney and spag bol, and comfort-food and comfort-sex are both great things, but they are emotionally distinct from fine food and fantastic sex, both of which are generally enjoyed in public places amongst kindred spirits ...'

'Though they're too rich for everyday consumption,' put in Johnny, 'and probably simply for most metabolisms including mine. Just not Mark's, though ...'

And in truth, I have known many chefs and food critics who are privileged daily to eat the finest and rarest ingredients, but I have yet to encounter one who has lost the capacity to enjoy – or to appreciate the significance of – a bowl of champ, or a home-cooked hotpot.

So, too, I have never met a swinger who no longer enjoys sex with his or her partner because of their shared adventures with others. On the contrary, visits to restaurants and forays into swinging both seem to stimulate appetite and inventiveness at home.

Cheap fast food guzzled on the hoof simply to assuage hunger is, like casual sex, altogether another matter – just sad, abusive, unhealthy and unworthy.

4

THE NASTIEST OBJECTION OF ALL ...

AND SO TO THE NASTIEST of all objections to swinging – the last refuge of the fascist who seeks to express disapproval whilst retaining putative liberal kudos. Like all truly vile arguments for constraints of freedom, this too takes an aesthetic form. These are the aesthetics of arrogance and intolerance.

I consulted the Internet and visited the library for written accounts of swinging. Again and again, journalists who 'exposed' the scene – as though it were a secret freemasonry, rather than a subculture open to anyone with a few pounds in his pocket – expressed distaste for the bodies or the age of those whom they had observed at play.

Suppose that a commentator were to write of a gay couple that, whilst their desires were acceptable and their affection charming, their sexual activities were disgusting because they were not in the first flush of youth and their bodies were sagging and wrinkled.

Any editor worthy of the name would dismiss such a hack out of hand. Even in reviewing a public show, where – perhaps – it were more justifiable in that the audience pays for the pleasure of watching, any halfway decent commentator would surely hesitate to impute that a performer should desist on the grounds of cellulite or age.

Yet journalists routinely deride swingers for being ordinary people with ordinary bodies, rather than glamour models and porn-stars.

Astonishingly, it is the publications that drool most admiringly over the sexual antics of rock and celluloid divinities that sneer most repulsively at mere mortals for presuming to enjoy similar pleasures.

In what other context would a supposedly impartial commentator be permitted to write of 'lumpy, misshapen bodies going at it' or 'men with jiggle bellies and flaccid cocks getting to work on a pair of lady galumphers with hanging arses and stretch marks'?

If this was about a middle-aged wedding, a sporting event or an amateur dramatics production, this would correctly be perceived as grossly offensive bad journalism, revealing far more of the writer than of his purported subject. Because it is about a party at Colette's in New Orleans (a swingers' club, where I have enjoyed several delightful evenings) such offensive drivel is published without question or cavil.

Is there the least moral distinction between such irrelevant imposition of arbitrary and arrogant aesthetics and, for instance, racism or prejudice against the disabled? If so, I certainly cannot see it. Or is sexual pleasure, in this commentator's world, restricted to those with fame, money and surgically enhanced physiques?

Some swingers, I was to discover, are beautiful by any conventional standards. Some at whom we might not have spared more than a passing glance when upright and clothed prove beautiful by reason of their vulnerability, their sassy confidence, their passion and the sparkle in their eyes when naked and ecstatic. Some are decidedly physically unlovely – by my standards.

But my standards have nothing to do with it.

Yes, occasionally I have shuddered at the mountains of juddering, goose-pimpled flesh or at the shrivelled husks of bodies at certain parties, but at the same time I confess to admiration for, and sympathy with, those who nonetheless have the pride to play in defiance of a world still more judgemental than that which condemns the rest of the subculture.

5

SEX = IMMORALITY

AGAIN AND AGAIN, I was to discover that it was not the circumstances or the consequences of sex but simply sex itself (or rather
sexual pleasure; dutiful, wearisome sex appeared immune from censure) that was associated with immorality.

This is no doubt the legacy at once of the notion that sex invariably means penetration and ejaculation, and so conception, and of
the infantile conflation of inaccessibility or prohibition and naughtiness.

The former was irrelevant. It seemed to me that the true moralist
(I speak here not of the sorry fantasist who would construct morality
for humans upon the premiss that we might or should be insubstan-
tial spirit, but rather of him who would work human clay to its finest
forms) should be concerned with the means whereby sex might best
be enjoyed and celebrated without doing harm – not with its denial.

As for the latter, whilst all play is of its nature 'naughty' – irresponsible, daring, frivolous, 'ludicrous' – I was no more willing to consider
the greatest of all sensual pleasures and of inspirations to poetry and

art a smutty, degenerate pastime, because of childish misunderstanding and fear, than I was about to devote half the Christmas budget to rebuilding the chimney for Santa.

Lisa, who parked her wagon in a field 500 yards away on her visits, sometimes watched daytime television. One day, we saw a singularly ugly woman there. She was, of course, relating the tales of her misfortunes. She said that she had once made a living as a 'clip artist' – one who posed as a prostitute, took a fee in advance from would-be clients, then ran away, providing no service in exchange for her fee.

'Of course, I wasn't going to *do* them,' she said smugly. 'I never lost my morals. I got my self-respect.'

This preposterous assertion passed unchallenged. Her listeners nodded. There was even a patter of applause.

Here was a woman avowing that she had been an exploitative cheat and thief, occasioning untold distress to those who had entered into a contract with her in good faith. Yet she regarded herself as morally acceptable (and, by implication, honest prostitutes who rendered service in exchange for a fee as 'immoral') and retained 'self-respect' because her sorry genitals had remained inviolate.

That is how far we have sunk into the association of 'morality' with a peculiar, proscriptive notion of sexual probity.

If Mother Theresa had had a penchant for occasional adventures involving bondage or multiple partners, she would, *de facto,* have been irredeemably 'immoral'. If a liar and cheat who has contributed nothing to the total of human happiness professes herself sexually useless, she is thereby redeemed.

Many newspapers have so far profited from this absurd conflation that they regularly 'expose' people's harmless consensual sexual practices, so causing irreparable hurt to their families and friends, whilst purporting to perform a 'moral' function. Sex is 'immoral', so victimisation and intrusion assume the guise of morality.

Worse still, on the dubious principle that he who renounces pleasure is *de facto* morally superior to others (whence the respect afforded to vegetarians and ascetic but useless saints), any man – and most certainly any woman – who acknowledges enjoyment of sex without conventional sanction thereby loses credibility.

• • •

So far as I can now discern from three years' experience, there is little that can be branded 'immoral' in contemporary swinging.

'Amoral' is quite another matter, but the word presupposes that all sex should, of its nature and regardless of context, be a moral matter.

Where there are resultant attachments and obligations involved, so, of course, it is. Where, however, we are talking about strangers pursuing mutual pleasure and explicitly committed to remaining unattached – at least to one another – to contraception, to courtesy and to safe sex, this is not so obvious.

Remove from sex the grave consequences which made it a life-changing, life-creating, life-destroying act. Separate it from the emotions and obligations inevitably surrounding such an act. Can we then enjoy it for itself as a life-asserting, liberating, ecstatic, communicative and companionable experience?

A glance at many of the world's societies, at our primate cousins and at our own people in youth, shows that many – if not all of us – can and do. The concept of sex as 'sacred' and exclusive is neither essential nor instinctive, but merely the product of social constructs and consequent economic necessities.

Many of those constructs still remain in law and in tabloid morality, and, of course, in much of our literature and our customs. Over the past fifty years, however, with contraception reliable and women financially empowered, the circus wagons appear to have broken down and the more spirited animals have broken out of their cages and run on, often confused and scared (sometimes even savage) ahead.

Again this is not to question the potential for sex to express a very particular love and commitment, nor to deny the value of such commitments. Both are fundamental tenets of swingers' ethics. We are all surely aware, however, that this is not sex's sole function.

Unlike much of the routine sex of conventional marriage and relationships founded upon convenience or personal advantage unrelated to sexual desire (curious, that the people who most fervently sing of the searing flame of romantic love as the sole justification for sex are also the principal champions of dutiful contentment amidst its clinker), swinging sex is always desired by both or all parties.

Emancipated woman has broken free of lifelong hire-purchase whoredom. Her transition to sensuous wantonness by choice – to anything by choice – is surely desirable.

Unlike the 'love' affairs that break up politicians' families, yet mysteriously win the sympathy of otherwise censorious tabloids because 'love' is posited, swingers' long-term relationships tend to be stable and their adventures – if gregarious – courteous and discreet. Swingers' children, business-partners and 'straight' friends generally remain unaware of their hobby.

Unlike the febrile fumblings and jerkings of teenage clubbers, swinging has strictly enforced protocols ensuring mutual respect and sexual hygiene.

Unlike the commonplace and grotesque parade/charades of wine-bars and drinks parties, there is no ambivalence or deception in swingers' seduction, little chance of one partner expecting romance or commitment whilst the other is driven only by sexual urges. The ambiguities and the power-struggles that characterise one-on-one sexual relationships are renounced by swingers, to whom explicitness and mutuality are prerequisites.

It was easy enough for me, as a liberally educated countryman, to accept sex as a gift of the gods and not, of its nature, ugly or immoral. I was surprised, however, to find not a single utilitarian objection to swinging *vis à vis* its more conventional vanilla alternatives.

6

THE VANILLA ONE-NIGHT STAND

I CONSIDERED THOSE ALTERNATIVES. Aside from marriage or long-term commitment – which was not only prohibited for me, but must be at best self-deceptive and hurtful – there was only the standard, squalid, exploitative (all right, often mutually exploitative, but little the better for that) one-night stand.

I had many experiences of these. They tended to be unsatisfactory. Their emotional duration, for at least one participant, seldom endured for just one night.

Annabel is a friend of Lisa's – a thirty-three-year-old mother-of-two and an occasional swinger. She gave me the following appraisal of commonplace 'vanilla' one-night stands:

'Like most modern girls, I've had them. And, like most of my friends, I've found them OK but, yeah, sort of sad.

'I mean, first, the sex is usually moderate. You have to be pretty good to suss one another out – what you like, what is allowed, what your fantasies are – first time, and usually after an evening of tension and posturing and drinking too much.

'So it's generally an urgent, clumsy sort of reconnaissance in which you're both out to get what you can, and both of you are left feeling unfulfilled, impersonal and dissatisfied. Neither has given a good account of him- or herself. It's all to do with need, nothing to do with celebration.

'And the one-night stand uses the same language as love – all those secretive smiles and little trying-it-out caresses, the gifts and intimate revelations, the expressions of hopes and sadnesses and fears. When all that is over, perhaps you can both admit that you're actually looking for an otherwise meaningless shag, but by then the emotional imbalance is guaranteed.

'And it's intimate. I don't mean the sex. I mean the tooth brushing and teddy bears and your side of the bed, water or cigarettes on the bedside table, telephones and alarm-clocks, clothes folded neatly or just flung down in blobs on the floor. A bedroom is a private place. Bedtime has its private rituals.

'When I'm in another person's room, I must take in his or her memories and taste in books, pictures, furnishings and a thousand other things. When he or she is in mine, it's the same thing. It's my family photographs and the CDs I'm a bit embarrassed about, and my make-up and knickers scattered around the room. It's an invasion.

'Hotels are worse, if anything. Luggage is as intimate as it gets, and the morning after, there's the clean impersonality of the room, the condoms like twisted slugs on the carpet, the scattered towels and clothes. They just underline the futility of all that "darling" stuff and all that snogging and panting.

'And really one-night stands are very masculine things. By the nature of sexuality and its conventions – whether he's in my house or I'm in his – I have to accept his masculinity whilst he has to make almost no concession to me. A hotel may put chocolates on the pillow and throw in a hairdryer and a couple of carnations, but it's always a functional, masculine thing, and the male after a one-night stand has to get dressed in an identity. The old role of the swaggering male who has "scored" is hanging there ready for him.

'I mean, I may have "scored" too, but I can't dress up in that. Why would I? Why would getting fucked by one male out of millions be something to be proud of?

'When I'm playing, though, the whole thing's on my terms as much as – if not more than – on his. We're on neutral territory designed to afford what are always thought of as female pleasures – sexy clothes, lush décor, soft lighting, crappy music, a drink in the hand, the caresses of warm water and attractive women, the powerful turn-on of other people having fun all about you – and there's no pressure. If I feel like it, I can do nothing but chat and watch, or I can beckon to one man or woman out of twenty, then turn away from him or her when I've had enough or when another one takes my fancy.

'Men and women are equals here, equally seeking fun and sensory pleasure and, at the end of it all, we dress and walk away having lost nothing. There's just desire – or not – not need or loneliness. There's no invasion of privacy or intimacy, just sex and sensuality, and it's all celebration rather than purging. And let's face it, the reason we have one-night stands, and the reason that they are one night, is that we want a shag. Face up to that and you can start going about it more logically, more safely and more joyfully.

'I've never left a swingers' party where I've played, without feeling pride and a nice warm sense of satisfaction. And I can honestly look back on them all with pleasure. I can't think of a single one-night stand of which I can say the same.'

7

SWINGING AND HEALTH

I TURNED, THEN, FROM theoretical to practical concerns.

The health risks of swinging, it seemed, were small.

'Oh, Lord, no. Swingers are like prostitutes,' Johnny assured me. 'They're generally much safer than the sexually active public,because they expect to be having sex with strangers. So they take precautions in advance and demand that their partners do, and there's none of that, "Oo-er, the passion was too much for us. Fuck the risk" stuff that I get from my patients all the time.

'Technically, I suppose, there is a very small risk from unprotected oral sex with multiple partners, but it is negligible unless you have major oral lesions. And, from what I can gather, swinging men don't often come in women's mouths. Overall, and subject to all the usual cautions, I'd say you were safer there than in ordinary, single, sexually active civvy life.'

This left just one danger, and – as an addict – it is one of which I am acutely aware.

With most pleasures, there is a law of diminishing returns. I was scared that orgiastic sex with multiple strangers might render all other sexual experiences tame and uninteresting, and would demand ever wilder extremes.

Lisa reassured me. As far as she was concerned at least, there was room for different varieties of sex. 'This is fantasy, like the fantasies you have when you're masturbating – which can be pretty crazy and nasty, but actually only stimulate you when you're back home making love with one person. I mean, unless you're seriously ill, your fantasies of being forcibly fucked by a whole regiment don't affect your enjoyment of sex with your nearest and dearest, do they?

'It's like the classical musician getting off on a night in the disco. You're saying the same things but in different ways. Most swingers are in long-term relationships and have very busy sex lives together. I suppose it could happen, but the two things are just so different.'

• • •

I vowed to myself that I would remain alert to the possibility. I have done so.

And yes, swinging sex proves one of those appetites that grows by what it feeds on, but it is an appetite for more kisses, more caresses, more sensual pleasures, more distinctive tastes and characteristic responses, more fun – not greater degrees of excess. Swinging sex has increased my appetite for – and, I hope, my proficiency in – more discreet and exclusive sexual communication.

Astonishingly, despite the apparently general assumption that swinging was, somehow, obscurely morally wrong, I could find not a single valid ethical objection to it.

I look forward to hearing of one that I missed.

8

'I WAS BORN NAKED IN EDEN, WASN'T I?'

NOT ONLY, THEN, DID SWINGING SEEM to be safe and at worst morally neutral, but, according to Lisa, swingers enjoyed their hobby only subject to strict rules.

Sir Francis Dashwood and his consciously rebellious, debauched friends in the Hellfire Club borrowed as the motto for their orgies Rabelais's '*Fay Ce Que Vouldra*' or 'Do what you will'.

Such anarchy, it seemed, is far removed from the ethos of modern swinging.

Dashwood's blasphemous orgies were fuelled (like their religious predecessors) by alcohol, drugs and incantation, and most of its female participants were prostitutes. But drunkenness is almost unknown at swingers' parties, drugs – but for the odd joint out in the garden – are strictly forbidden, and working girls attend – if at all – only for a busman's holiday.

'They're just straight social occasions,' Lisa shrugged. 'Meetings, greetings, gossip ... Aside from the playrooms – and okay, the sometimes crazy, OTT costumes – the only thing that distinguishes them from vanilla drinks parties is the ease with which subjects that most people think of as threatening or difficult are openly discussed."

She was right there. Swingers' conversation can seem startling when written down. Overheard from last night: 'We really wanted to play with them but I got my period the very evening we arrived ...' 'Oh, yes, we played with them – when was it, darling? Couple of months ago? That cock is terrifying!' 'Silly sod got so excited he came all over this new dress. I was like, "Oh, that's good ... No! Help! Christ!", diving behind the sofa for cover. I could have killed him.' But when you hear it, it's so easy, so unaffected, so untainted by exhibitionism or connivance, that it might as well be fellow-golfers talking about courses.

'The thing I love is that there's no hidden sexual agenda here,' Annabel told me. 'Just for once, men and women, in front of their partners, can touch, kiss or express appreciation of other people without causing jealousy, or having to hide their sexual feelings beneath banter or allusion.

'Swinging couples might enjoy a conversation and become friends but never consider having sex, or they could reject one another's proposals of sex without causing any resentment.'

'You'll enjoy it,' said Lisa. 'Stop fussing. It's just good, clean fun ...' And then, when I raised my eyebrows, she added, 'Yeah, well, it *is* clean. It's uncluttered and untainted by all the world's usual prejudices, fears and emotional complications.

'It's clean (and, okay, mucky) like rugby is clean – and battle is anything but. Swingers play just like children do – no expectations, inhibitions, imposed responsibilities, status. Even stereotypical sexual identities – gay, bi, straight, sub, dom, etc. – go by the board really. You just frolic in a fantasy world.

'The reason the story of the Fall works so well is that we all do it, we all feel it,' Lisa went on. 'So, like at puberty, we taste forbidden fruit and are chucked out of Eden, and from then on we're meant to be tainted and guilty. Whole areas of our bodies are taboo. All physical play from say thirteen onwards has to be cautious and inhibited, especially nowadays when the law has a mind as dirty as any perv. If it does inspire sexual response, we're meant to feel ashamed.

'So swingers, like us, think, "Hang on. I was born naked in Eden, wasn't I? A naked princess in Eden. It's my birthright. Why should my natural sexuality debar me? What jumped up arsehole says so?" As far as we're concerned, it was the shame, not the tasting, that was the original sin. We aim to take our sexuality back into Eden, say "Fuck you" to those who don't like it, and frolic and play proudly just like when we were children.

'And everywhere else, it's sort of adult concerns that decide who you fuck, like money, social background and how they're dressed and ... This is sex as a game, not a lasting social commitment. So you play with people of all backgrounds, people you might have nothing in common with in other circumstances, but here you're united by just humanity, sensuality and acceptance of both in others. You don't enquire into their race, wealth or social rank, just, "Is he or she fanciable and will he or she give a lot and have a laugh?"'

Caroline, 42, an estate agent acquaintance of Lisa's, agreed. 'God, the number of men and women I've seen in my life and I've thought, "Ooh, I'd do them if only it weren't for their table-manners, or way of talking, or the idea of finding them there in the morning!"

'But in the Lifestyle, all that goes out of the window. You can play with them because you're both raunchy and they are pretty and have nice smiles, and it can be beautiful and warm and affectionate and – "Thanks, love, that was great and bye, bye". No need to worry about anything else.

'You go to a party. The welcome's always warm. The jokes are uninhibited. Everyone's kind and affectionate. And when the game is over, swingers go back to their normal, everyday identities and duties.'

Much is made today of avoidance of commitment. 'He (or, less commonly, she) is afraid of commitment' is generally used as an insult. It is seldom considered that avoidance of commitment might actually be desirable, intelligent and considerate, and that more grief is caused by commitments irresponsibly made – or assumed to be made – on the grounds of sexual attraction, than was ever caused by sex for its own sake.

'Swingers can be attracted, have sex with someone and move on,' said Lisa, 'or, after sex, become their close friends, where everywhere else, relationships seem to be ordained simply by the fact of sex, whether it be good, bad or indifferent, and all the expectations and obligations, affections or guilty animosities arising from that fact.'

Swingers almost invariably refer to their hobby as 'playing'. It is a word well chosen. War is dangerous and has many casualties. We therefore play games on sports fields in order to indulge the impulses which give rise to – and which spring from – war, but we play them only in public and subject to strict rules.

Swinging (and sex too has many casualties) seems to be playing in the same sense. Just as rugby players hate one another only during the game and then afterwards retire to the bar for a drink, just as children desire the deaths of their enemies as they fire their fingers at them, then go home to share jellies and to pass-the-parcel, so – as Stevie Nicks relates – 'Players only love you when they're playing.'

Afterwards, although the shared experience creates a bond, swingers return to their other lives and responsibilities.

'The other frustrated fantasists indulging their whims are just playing unregulated war-games with real weapons,' said Caroline, 'and real weapons tend to have lives of their own and to fulfil their natures despite all the best intentions of those brandishing them.'

All in all – and yes, I acknowledge that I wanted to think thus, but this made it harder, not easier to believe – I really could not discern a single reason why I should not give swinging a whirl.

Lisa had been growing increasingly frustrated with me as I questioned all and sundry as to their views.

Now I yielded. 'OK,' I announced. 'I want this. Let's do it.'

PART III

1

INVITATION TO AN ORGY

IF THIS WERE A PORNOGRAPHIC MEMOIR, I could devote the whole of it to encounters and orgies on the British swing-scene, which would doubtless be of passing interest to a certain sort of reader in the heat of sexual desire or frustration, but would repel the sated and, at length, bore even the wanker.

This is not, as some will claim, because every encounter is the same and that orgies and participants meld into an amorphous blur. One could as well argue that every steeplechase, say, is trivial and forgettable, or every fine meal indistinguishable from another. It is simply untrue. A word, a name, a scent is sufficient to conjure each individual race or meal in all its brilliant intensity. And the principal joy of swinging sex is precisely that each new partner is wonderfully, excitingly different.

For all that, a book which described steeplechase after steeplechase, dinner after dinner, must soon become monotonous. This is not a fault of the things described, but of our vocabulary and the terms of reference at our disposal with which to describe pleasure or, for that matter, pain.

Caressing, kissing, licking, sucking, fucking – this is the basic, tawdry syntax of sex, just as boiling, frying, grilling and roasting are the terms with which we describe the core functions of the cook.

They are just technical terms which tell us nothing of the infinite subtleties ordained on the one hand by the individual people, moods and circumstances, on the other by the peculiar nature of the ingredients and the facilities on offer.

Cooking admits of minor distinctions – simmering, sauteeing and the like – but recipes do not begin to describe the subtleties and occasional glories of great food, lovingly prepared in the right context. Our attempts to do just that therefore tend to use metaphor and simile which alienate and obscure rather than enlighten.

So I have a choice. I could attempt to describe in factual, actuarial terms the hundred or so orgies that I have attended in the past three years, and the couples whom I have met at my home – or at theirs – with a view to sexual adventure, and so bore rather than cajole the pants off the reader. Or I could wax as lyrical as each such event deserves, which might be of momentary interest to the wanker, but would fail to convey either information or a sense of the feelings involved to anyone save myself.

Let's go, then – for now at least – to just one swingers' party.

Let's go – for the sake of honesty and in order to obviate any blaseness which I may unwittingly have acquired – to my first such party, where I feigned assurance but gazed about me with all the incredulous delight of, say, Tom of the *Water Babies* transported to Disneyland, or Cinderella at last arriving at the palace.

2

A CINDERELLA WITH A FUCK-CARD

I HAD – IN THE COURSE of a normal vanilla life – enjoyed just eight threesomes. In three of these, I had been one of two men with a girl. In the other five, I had been with two women. Oh, and there was a strange evening at my university where three female students asked their boyfriends – of whom I was one – to assist at a competition to establish which of them could come fastest. This led to inevitable protests that we males might have influenced the result, and so to exchanges of partners for non-penetrative sex.

Only one of those threesomes had been with people who thought of themselves as swingers.

I had also attended two wholesale orgies – one in Paris, when a student, and one more recently in Wimbledon, as the guest of an old friend. I was thirty-five, and Georgette had taken me along to observe. We separated at the door and went our own ways. I had sex with five women that night and fell passionately in love with each of them in turn. Three of them subsequently became friends and lovers.

Soon afterwards, however, I was in a long-term relationship, and – for all the interest that the experience had awoken in me – my swinging career was cut short.

Now, however, I was 47, divorced, and resuming where I had left off.

Our first swingers' party was in London's Docklands.

On the journey from the West Country, Lisa explained to me how swingers' parties work. They are, it seemed, a cross between the disco parties of my teenage years and the drinks parties and receptions of adulthood.

As at drinks parties, swingers meet – singly or in couples – form short-lived groups which absorb others, fragment and reform, and chatter a lot about the weather, sport, their sex lives, the cost of living, their possessions, their children and the government.

As at the teenage party, where communication is generally limited to hair patting, sneering and preening followed by a bit of mutual gut wriggling, the intention of the whole business is manifest if largely unstated. At teenage parties the dance floor slowly empties as couple after couple retires into dark corners to slobber over one another, and to fondle one another's crevices. Here too, couple after couple will drift off into the playrooms, remove their clothes and 'play'.

'Generally, you play with one another,' explained Lisa, 'and then others come and join you, or people playing on the bed or mattress beside you begin touching you and checking out your response. Maybe you like them and swap with them, or play as a foursome for a while. So, say you've got a girl sitting on a guy's cock and the other girl's sitting on his face and sucking the other guy or whatever. And then another couple is playing nearby, and one of you reaches out to stroke her or kiss him, and so it goes on ...'

But few swingers spend an entire evening in the thick of the action. 'You need a break – food, drink, a piss, even just a rest – so you go off into the social rooms again. And that's the second way of meeting people you play with. You're there – naked or just dressed in underwear or something – and you meet some people and like them, and one of you will say, "Shall we go and play?" so you all pile back in together and the whole thing starts all over again.

'Of course, you may have no interest in the others playing around you. That's cool,' Lisa shrugged, 'you just play with one another. Other people come along; you just shake your head, say "No, thanks."'

Most couples, she told me – again as at drinks parties – attend as couples and won't be separated. 'Some couples will just stick together for the first hour or so then split up, just coming back from time to time to check that the other one's OK ...'

In many ways, then, the swingers' party seemed to me to resemble the more conventional sort of ball, with fucking at last taking its rightful throne from that unconvincing pretender, dance. The chatter, the introductions, the proposals accepted or rejected, the 'excuse me's', the set-piece communal dances, the timorous 'wallflowers' – even the conga – all find their echoes in the modern orgy.

Lisa, a Georgette Heyer fan, liked this allusion. 'Yeah. Quite fancy the idea of a fuck-card attached to my wrist: "May I have the honour of the 10.30 sixty-nine, or the midnight slow fuck?" "La, sir! But we barely know each other! Perhaps a well-lit blow-job would be more appropriate ..." But yeah, basically, you've got the idea.'

3

THE WARM-UP

THE DOCKLANDS PARTY WAS reassuringly small, and run by a trio of city business types who call themselves 'Coupleszone'. The location of their regular orgies changed from month to month, but it was usually a luxurious flat or house somewhere within the square mile.

This was a 'Couples Only' party. Many clubs and swingers' groups permit a limited number of single males to enter on specific nights. Some men's enthusiasm flags in the course of the evening, whilst women's tends to remain constant or to increase with each adventure. These single men, therefore, provide a reserve energy supply. The usual convention in the clubs is that males are permitted on Friday nights, but only couples on Saturdays.

The extent of selectivity imposed at each venue varies widely. At the better clubs – such as Chameleons in Birmingham and at Liberations in Leicester – single males must submit photographs and lengthy forms before they are considered, and must then remain on a waiting list for a long while before they will be admitted. Other clubs are less stringent in their requirements, particularly since single males must pay up to three times the entrance fee paid by couples. Single females, unsurprisingly, are always welcome.

Most of these clubs also have 'Greedy Girls' nights in their calendars. At these, the single males (who again pay a great deal for the privilege) outnumber the women by a factor of three or more to one.

Lisa and I travelled to London by train. I had booked into one of those supersonic, globetrotting hotels whose foyers boast acres of textured MDF panels, a great deal of curious lighting and 100-yard reception desks, staffed by one woman in a cardboard-cut-out suit and jabot and one man with a yellow tie. Piped music – like light – seeped and puddled into this vast space and dribbled from invisible speakers into the pill-capsule lift.

Our room was a box with a huge window overlooking the Thames. Our bed was also a large, hard box. It did not matter. As Lisa said, 'With any luck, we'll be returning totally shagged at four in the morning, so who cares? It's clean, isn't it?'

This is a sound and thrifty principle for swingers. Luxury suites are wasted.

She showered and enjoyed dressing up. This is always one of the most pleasurable and most childlike aspects of swinging. Women can indulge their every last 'look at me' fantasy of sweeping staircases, stilettos, thigh-high boots, slashed skirts or no skirt, glittering panties or no panties, satin, lace, leather, PVC or liquid latex. Some content themselves with lavish corsets or plain little black dresses. The only article of clothing that appears *de rigueur* is stockings – whether hold-ups or sustained with suspenders.

Some enjoy fancy dress, and there are usually a few French maids, cowgirls, traffic-cops and the like in the mix. Lisa dressed simply that night. Her bra, thong and hold-up stockings were lemon yellow. She wore a short, black, accordion-pleated skirt and a scoop-yoked golden silken top with a parrot and jungle foliage design. Ferragamo – via Oxfam.

I wore what would become my swinging uniform – black velvet evening slippers, black silk socks, plain black trousers, a white poplin shirt with gold links, and an off-the-peg blue blazer.

I had thought carefully about this outfit. I retain it to this day because my reasoning still seems sound.

On the one hand, I need to carry a pen (for names and numbers), cards, cigarettes and at least twenty condoms (some parties and clubs have bowls of free condoms in every room, but many rely on you to bring your own), and I am sufficiently fogeyish to want to make an effort – at least in part – to match that made by the women in their sparse but sexy finery.

On the other, I was and am well aware that these clothes will – with luck – be worn for a short time only, and will spend the greater part of the evening crumpled and frequently trampled where they fall. A swingers' party is not the place for your fragile Sunday best.

I removed all credit cards from my coat and retained just £60 in cash in my back pocket. It is unlikely that there will be petty thieves about – nor have I met any since then – but there seems no point in taking the risk, or putting temptation in anyone's way.

Lisa and I then learned spontaneously a regular and delicious feature of preparation for parties. As she raised a foot onto the armchair to lace her golden sandals, I dived in there and we played for fifteen minutes or so, which meant she had to rearrange her make-up and hair.

Since then, I have dressed for hundreds of parties with many different women. We have always played together as part of the process. Sometimes, when we have guests round, I have played with as many as five girls in turn and together before setting off.

This is the warm-up, the *amuse-gueule*, the delicious equivalent of the freshly baked bread, the Negroni, the sussuration of linen and the tattoo of cutlery and glass. It is an essential part of the fun.

4

DRESSING TO UNDRESS

PLAY CONTINUED IN THE mini-cab. The driver, inevitably, got lost and asked us for directions. We were amused, then irritated.

At length, after two calls to our hosts, we found ourselves at the electronic gates of a residential riverside block.

We were buzzed into a hall lined with green brocade. The console tables were gilt, with marble tops. The chandelier was of giant Bohemian teardrops. The lift – for some strange reason in a building so plainly modern – was of the double gate, lattice variety.

We were warmly greeted by a man in his mid-thirties. He was slim and well spoken. His sandy hair was receding, his chin of the sort with which furrows could be ploughed. His smile, however, carved a broad diamond on his face. His teeth were dazzling. Lisa plainly liked him.

The girl beside him was a little younger. Her hair was short and blonde. Her eyes were blue and bright. She wore a clinging, dark blue jersey frock with a plunging bodice and a skirt that covered her

· knees. She kissed both of us on both cheeks. They could have been any prosperous couple welcoming us to spag-bol dinner with friends.

Behind them, there was the usual rumble and chatter of a drinks party. Carl and Angie showed us around and introduced us to a few couples as we went.

The guests were dressed conventionally enough. Here or there a skirt was slit to the hip. One woman wore PVC boots which snaked to mid-thigh. Another wore sandals like Lisa's – laced, Greek-style, up the calf. Skirts might, on average, be a little shorter than usual – one was short enough to show stocking-tops – bodices cut a little lower, trousers a little rarer, but few people here would have looked out of place at a contemporary cocktail bar.

The men were the usual confused mess denoted by the words 'smart casual'. Their shirts and, no doubt, their trousers, were expensive and well pressed. There was no obviously man-made fibre on view. The shirts, however, flapped loose. The deck shoes and trainers seemed out of place.

OK. To a fogey.

• • •

Women's choice of dress at swingers' parties is, I was to learn, constrained by just one factor which may not be so pressing for others – the ease with which garments may be removed and, rather more important, put back on.

Although she will strip off to play, a female swinger will then want to rejoin the throng outside the playrooms. Few like to do so totally naked. Intricate lace-up corsets or basques may be popular amongst beginners, but they are therefore rare amongst more experienced players, who generally favour expensive but mechanically simple underwear and dresses.

Boots and shoes are the exception. Because swinging women tend

to wear stockings, they need not remove their intricate and fanciful ·
footwear when they undress. This makes for a delightful but sometimes alarming spectacle. I have often knelt on a mattress with
stiletto heels flailing at groin level, their owners blissfully unaware of
the nose-cutting, face-spiting dangers that they pose.

Vanessa – a friend who came down from Warwickshire with her
husband, Simon, to stay with us for a swinging weekend – spent an
entire Saturday night party itching to join the action. But, having
played soon after our arrival, then having had Simon, me and my
swing-partner take twenty minutes to lace her up again, could not
bring herself to go through the whole laborious process all over
again.

Of course, not every woman feels the need to dress after playing.
Some enjoy the freedom of strutting their stuff and wandering about
the party unclothed. Many, however, for peculiarly feminine reasons,
choose not to be entirely naked. Sally, for example, always wore a
thin gold chain around her belly. 'I can't explain it. All the bits that
I'm meant to be worried about are on show, and it feels great, but that
silly little chain just means that I'm wearing something which is
mine. Weird, but there it is.'

Some private parties are – usually unoriginally – themed: Roman
Orgy, Tarts and Vicars, Schooldays, Fetish … With very few exceptions, such themes can be ignored. They are opportunities for silli-
ness and aids to playfulness, not requirements.

● ● ●

There were two couples here who might be in their mid-twenties.
There were three who might be in their late forties or early fifties.
The average age, however, must be around thirty-five to forty-five.
No one here was overweight.

Neither of us wanted alcohol, so we had brought ten bottles of ginger beer and, as a gauche – considering we were paying £25 admission – contribution to our hosts, a bottle of champagne. These were placed in the fridge in the kitchen. We were led back through the big living room with its balcony overlooking the river, then to the left again, into two bedrooms. Tonight, they were playrooms. The beds took up 90 per cent of the available space.

We returned to the living room and chatted, first to one of the older couples – she, tall, blonde, tanned, slightly gaunt, in training for the London Marathon, he, shorter, smooth, with slicked-back greying dark hair and a slow, one-sided salesman's smile. They holidayed at a naturist colony on the Isle of Wight and on their yacht which was moored in Torquay. Next week they were off to a swingers' resort in Cancun, Mexico.

Then came a younger foursome – the girls looking mildly ill at ease, the men falsely confident, limber and flash in their brilliant, open-necked shirts.

Then a girl whom I particularly liked – a dark bob, strong dark features, a long, beautiful body in a swooping black dress with a slit skirt. She was an American academic, her subject the seventeenth-century English stage. He was a banker, but they were not here to play, they said, merely to observe. They had had some experience of the scene in Chicago, but had only heard rumours of the London swing-set. This was their first foray.

Then a French girl, early thirties, tiny, trim, bright and bumptious – 'Hello, I am the bouncering person. May I have your name please?' – with a remarkably good looking husband – curly brown hair and an athlete's body. He was an artist – formerly in the British army – she, a mother-of-two ...

But, interesting and congenial though all this was, it was the eyes that did the talking, not merely with those with whom we chatted, but with many others about the room.

• • •

Perhaps it always is. At a straight drinks party too, we appraise with our eyes, approving, dismissing, interested, amused, desiring, but aware that we are likely to meet only a few of those whom we see.

Eye contact is brief, decorous and frequently broken off out of fear. Just occasionally, our flickering gazes are drawn into a long, lingering, lip-licking maelstrom. Occasionally they are flung back with a mocking *moue* and a cock of the hips. In general, however, they pass – no doubt noticed but unacknowledged – the loose change of human transactions.

Here, physical assessments were mirrored, smiles congenially returned. Glances were still fleeting, but they were frankly acknowledged. Later, we would all meet, or at least see one another, without these defensive clothes and manners.

Time and again at such parties, I have observed a woman amidst the crowd, the 'cut of whose jib' – as my father would say – pleases me. My glance has passed over her, and has been cursorily, inexpressively returned, but that merest split second longer than would be normal in the vanilla world.

Initially, I took this for dismissal, but invariably, in the thick of orgiastic action, it has been she who has lain down beside me, she who has crawled across a mattress to suck me when I am going down on another woman, she who has welcomed me into her arms, often, by now, aware of my name.

5

TIME TO PLAY

LISA HAD BY NOW HAD enough of conventional socializing. She unbuttoned her shirt, threw it down and languorously danced to the music – now Getz and Gilberto.

I was frankly nervous. 'Hey, hang on,' I said, looking over her shoulder at the impassive gazes of the others. 'No need to be impatient!'

She unhooked her skirt. It slithered to the floor. She stepped out of it and kicked it under the sofa. 'Why not?' she shrugged. In bra, thong and stockings, she sashayed up to me and linked her fingers at the nape of my neck. Her pelvis rotated against mine. 'I can't be doing with all this chuntering,' she said. 'We're here to play, aren't we? Let's play.'

She kissed me and, taking my hand, led me down the little corridor to the further bedroom.

There were already two couples in the half light. The Isle of Wight sailors were in a snuffling and clicking sixty-nine beneath the window. The lamplight from outside slicked them in shifting blue.

Closer at hand, a woman whom I had not noticed before – dark, glossy hair piled atop her head and escaping in artless curls down her cheeks – lay on her side. One foot was on the carpet, the other was up on the bed. She sucked the cock of a portly man lying on his back. Her shaven pussy was thus, inevitably, the part of her which first I met. It was very neat and pretty.

I stood by the bed. Lisa sat. She unzipped my flies and unfastened the waistband. I removed the blazer, unbuttoned my shirt and shrugged it off. As we played, her left hand caressed the thigh of the brunette at her side. I dropped to my knees to lick between Lisa's thighs. Following her lead, I too allowed my hand to creep up the brunette's stockinged thigh. Her pussy was welcoming. I slipped two fingers inside her. Her bent leg sank to allow me better access.

I knelt up to fuck Lisa, and still my fingers played with the other pussy at my right hand. Lisa's crown now rested on the portly man's hip. The brunette stopped sucking him to kiss her. I leaned over to kiss and suck on her nipples ...

Suddenly the bed and the floor all around it seemed filled with shifting bodies.

And so the fugue began.

6

GIUOCO DELLE COPPIE

I FIND IT DIFFICULT TO EXPLAIN how confused and kaleidoscopic are my memories of orgies.

This is not to say that the pictures which I retain are fuzzy. On the contrary, each is of heightened clarity – Lisa taking over from the Isle of Wight man in the sixty-nine with his wife, the brunette woman's husband asking me, 'Do you want to fuck her?', and my response to her, 'Do you want me to fuck you?', she smiling, nodding ...

Lisa now sucking two men, one over her shoulder, one before her face, whilst her entire body jerks from the fucking she is receiving from behind ...

Then she and I are playing together and she on her back as one of those young, confused-looking women approaches naked, and Lisa says luxuriantly, 'Oh, give me that!' and pouts up as the girl sinks into her arms ...

And then it is Lisa's turn to ask me 'Do you want to fuck her?' She has been crouching on her knees eating the girl for ten minutes as she asks me that. I tell her 'Yes,' and she grins. 'She's ready,' she says, three fingers still in the writhing girl's cunt. 'Oh, is she ready. Oh, are you ready ...' and she pulls me around her and into the girl and slaps my buttocks by way of encouragement ...

Time vanishes. Hours full of activity and excitement seem minutes. Somehow we are in the other bedroom, and two girls are crouched at my groin. Lisa joins them and pairs off with one of them whilst the other one straddles me, and the room is full of growling, panting, purring, yelping, squealing, humming, slapping bodies. There is joking too, and chatter, and a lot of kissing and soft moaning.

And then ... Then there is a moment of magic which seems to make the whole orgy freeze-frame. Lisa is leaving the bed to get a drink, and suddenly there is a tall, elegant woman of much the same age ahead of her, and the two women embrace and kiss – oh so deeply, oh so intimately – hands fluttering and grasping at one another's buttocks, backs and hair.

They sink to the bed together, still kissing, still caressing, totally focused, one on the other. They suck one another's fingers. They laugh softly into one another's mouths. They kiss one another's breasts and stomachs. They are wholly engrossed and so wholly engrossing. A space clears around them.

The girl with me is watching them as Lisa's head falls back onto my stomach and slowly the taller girl moves down her and laps between her legs. I stroke Lisa's hair and her head rocks slowly from side to side. Her eyes are closed. Her hips bob up and down, circle and, at the last, buck violently. She bites her knuckles and squeals through them. She rolls onto her side, clamping her thighs about the other girl's head, and the girl says 'Mmmm' and her eyes are wide and wondering.

Lisa has told me that she rarely comes at parties. This, it seems, is one of the exceptions.

Then it is Lisa's turn, and she too, with a hundred little, loving kisses, descends to the other girl's crotch. Again I supply – I am – the pillow, and the girl reaches up behind her head to grasp me as Lisa goes to work. Lisa's eyes are wide open now, watching her beloved's face as she nuzzles and licks into all that sweetness.

It is all outstandingly, bewilderingly beautiful.

The girl's boyfriend, who has thus far passed unnoticed, has pulled on a condom and now penetrates Lisa from behind. He is in his late thirties or early forties with a shaven head and well-developed pecs and arms. He frowns deeply, almost anxiously as he fucks.

He does not slam into Lisa, but fucks her slowly. The girls have ordained the rhythm to this dance. For all that, his intrusion has broken the spell. 'I was only fucking him out of politeness because I was fucking his wife,' Lisa shrugged afterwards, 'but you know, he was seriously good. I really enjoyed it.'

The bodies about us start to move again. The music breaks in on the reverie. At some point, the dark girl turns over and we play together. At some point, the play extends into the living room and even out onto the balcony, where my American academic friend so far forgets herself allowing her husband and me to play with her as she leans on the balustrade and gazes out over the corkscrew lights in the Thames.

I believe that battle is also usually recalled in this sort of crazy mosaic of memory.

Certainly there is sequentiality as each introductory kiss or caress leads onward, as each pairing or threesome or foursome splits and its components become players in new and different units.

Certainly too, for the detached observer, an orgy has its rhythms and a shape. Like a piece of music, it has its tranquil moments, its crescendi and diminuendi, its developments of particular themes. Different players step in to play their parts just as individual instruments enter to perform their own harmonic, melodic or contrapuntal functions.

As with music, the whole – notwithstanding thunderous climaxes, lyrical ensemble passages, innumerable scherzi and divers variations, improvisations and changes of tempo – aims so to build as to subsume individual consciousness until everyone present is caught up in its mood.

It is a very wonderful symphony.

7

INTERMEZZO INTERROTTO

BUT THEN, OF COURSE, this being life rather than music, it does not always work out. Sometimes an unexpected dissonance breaks the entire mood. Sometimes guests are dispirited or unwilling to participate so that the full ensemble is never achieved, and occasionally – this being human life – the fart of the tuba breaks in on the harmonies.

On this occasion, it took the form of a woman being 'spit-roasted' beside me. I was kneeling at the foot of a bed. A girl lay on her front facing me. The other woman was lying on her back at my right (so, perhaps I should say 'spit-fried', if such a thing existed). She was a middle-aged woman with frizzy colourless hair and perky little breasts topped by rose-pink nipples, which looked like plungers. She had bulging cabochon eyes, and bulging cabochon rings on every finger.

A man knelt at her head, thrusting his hips forward so that she could suck him. A dark man beside me knelt between her thighs and, leaning on straight arms, was fucking her with considerable enthusiasm. She said something like 'Hng' with his every thrust. When she stopped sucking, she snarled up at him, 'Yes! Fuck it! Fuck the little bitch! Go on, man! Stab it! Kill it!'

I could clearly see, then, her legs and his heaving buttocks and back, but these obscured my view of her upper torso and head. In general, when I saw her face, it was framed in a steep triangle between the man's left arm, his gleaming chest and her little breasts and ridged ribcage.

Suddenly she made a gargling sound. Her legs half straightened and started to shake so violently that her feet bounced clear of the bed's surface. I had seen that movement before.

The man between her legs evidently believed that his metronomic thrusting had worked elusive magic. He cried 'Yeah!' and 'Go on!' and jerked his hips fast and hard, a blissful smile now splitting his face. Sweat dripped from his brow and chest.

I now had a clear view of the woman. Her head was laid to one side, her jaw sagging, her lower lip lolling and wobbling, her eyes turned to marble. Close to orgasm, perhaps, but not close enough.

I reached over and tapped my neighbour on the shoulder. 'Er, hold it,' I said.

He turned his face to me. He wiped his brow on the back of his forearm and almost snarled. 'What? Yeah? What is it?'

'Just stop for a second, will you?'

'What? Why? What's up with you?'

'Just stop!' I barked so that heads turned. 'She's having a fit.'

'What you talking about?' His hips continued to shuttle back and forth. 'She's ...' he started. Then his arms flew up and he toppled sideways as I barged him clear.

I leaned forward and reached into the woman's mouth with forefinger and thumb. They emerged with her tongue between them, and a swooping, beaded string of saliva which did not break until my hand was back at the level of her stomach. I turned her into the recovery position.

The woman who had been at my groin was now kneeling naked at the woman's side. 'It's ... Hold on. I'm a nurse,' she said. She took the pulse whilst caressing the prone woman's flank – a professional caress, this one. She looked up at me. 'Hey, well spotted.' She turned to the man behind her. 'You're bloody lucky she didn't bite it off,' she told him coolly. 'Who's with her?'

'Oh, sorry ...' A naked man appeared in the doorway. He was small, bald and bespectacled, with a half-pint pot-belly. 'This has happened before. I think it's the heat ...'

'Yep. That'll do it, and the excitement,' the girl said as together we raised the woman's body, first to a sitting position, then to her feet. 'Has she seen a doctor?'

'No. She refuses. It only happens once in a while. You're all right, aren't you, Mags, girl?'

Mags drooled, ''m faaahn ... No problem ...' She lurched over her husband's shoulder so that her limp arm hung down almost to his navel.

'Take her out into the fresh air,' said my nurse friend. 'And take her to a doctor!' she called after the couple.

She leaned back against me.

'She OK?' I asked.

'She'll be fine. Syncope. Maybe epilepsy. I don't know. Bloody fool not to see someone about it, though.' My hand slid between her buttocks. She pushed backward against me.

The face which loomed close to mine was ugly. 'You didn't need to shove me!'

'Yes, he did,' said my new friend. 'Or did you want to shag a woman who wasn't even conscious?'

The man shrugged.

He actually shrugged.

'Jesus,' said the girl leaning against me. 'You are seriously *sick*.'

On other occasions, I have known a girl who contrived to get her foot caught between the slats of a bed-foot, whilst playing with three people at Swingers' Junction, and had to be released by the combined efforts of nine giggling, naked men and women. I have heard howls and yelps at attacks of cramp or back pain, or unexpected male ejaculation. I have also several times heard apologetic squeaks and whimpers as women ejaculated violently for the first time and believed that they had suddenly developed incontinence. Astonishingly, I have yet to witness or hear of a heart-attack.

8

'AFTER YOU'VE – YOU KNOW?'

ONE OF THE COMMONEST QUESTIONS that men are asked by non-swingers is, 'But what do you do after you've – you know?'

The questioner invariably looks bewildered when I answer that we seldom actually do 'you know'.

Swingers' parties are dedicated to luxury and erotic excitement, to prolonged sensory pleasure entailing sight, sound, scent, taste and touch. Orgasm – for the male at least – is an unnecessary and irritating interruption to such enjoyment. For thousands of male swingers, ejaculation is the special, private thing retained for a partner only. They 'save the last dance' for their special partners.

That first night, as on many since, I entered a state so erotically charged that I felt as though I were humming like a tuning-fork, and realised – without disappointment – that I had quite neglected to come.

Back in our hotel-room, Lisa and I attended to this matter and the result was so explosive that I was close to unconsciousness, as though drifting on a dark ocean beneath a star-sprinkled sky. The 'little death' seemed apt indeed.

I may have given a false impression in the account of this party in that I have written a lot about fucking. It so happens that there was a lot of coupling at this particular event. That is not inevitably the case.

The morning after that first night, I am ashamed to relate that I proudly totted up the number of women whom I had fucked, and with whom I had enjoyed oral sex. When I asked Lisa how many men and women she had fucked, she could not tell me. With some effort, she could tell me with how many people she had played. Fucking was just part of that process.

Reared in a phallocentric culture ('Did she go all the way?'), it took me a while to realise that fucking, if not irrelevant, is only one of many pleasurable sexual activities, and far from the most significant. Women seem to grasp this very rapidly.

Since that day I have discovered that most female swingers, unless profoundly disappointed, share Lisa's unconcern as to whether or not – in the course of play – fucking did or did not take place. 'It's just another form of play, and sometimes it's just what I need,' my swinging friend Laura told me, 'but, especially with condoms, it's just internal caressing along with external. I don't mean I'd like an evening of play without a fuck. I'd go crazy, but along the way it doesn't matter so much.'

My later swing-partner Sally left Utopia in Birmingham one night telling me, 'I hope you're wide awake, because you've got your work cut out tonight. I've played with God knows how many people and I've not been properly fucked once.' She had in fact played with three women and four men, two of whom turned out to be 'soft' swingers and two of whom had been more literally soft.

9

LESSONS LEARNED

I HAD LEARNED A LOT FROM this first experience.

First and foremost, I had learned that, for all my consideration in matters of dress, I was altogether inappropriately clad when naked.

Until the mid '90s, men remained hirsute. The only men who shaved then were body-builders, 'Chippendales' and their like, who exhibited their oiled torsos for money.

Well-groomed, sexually active women, meanwhile, had no body hair beyond neat, carefully topiaried arrowheads of pubic hair pointing to the bull. They trimmed the curls and went to the beautician for regular bikini-waxes. The less fortunate, fashion-conscious or fastidious left sprawling enravelments spreading outward almost to their thighs from a central black trunk which extended to their navels. The whole looked like a horse's tail, fully extended at the gallop, viewed from above.

My more recent infidelities had familiarised me with the 'Brazilian', which leaves only that trunk – albeit truncated – but lops off the branches, leaving a straight highway from the central belly to the labia.

I had only read of the 'Hollywood', or complete shave. But I always considered it mildly distasteful and associated it with men who, like Ruskin, preferred their women to look like statues or pre-pubescent girls.

Swingers, however, like the Imperial Romans, are shaven. Some leave a small dab of hair like a Hitler moustache. Some, like Lisa, leave a tonsure of fur only about the vagina itself. The majority are entirely hairless, though several have replaced their natural pelts with chicken-skin bumps, pimples or flushes of crimson in response to the blade. One woman at that London party, as if in honour of this effect, had orange and yellow flames tattooed across her entire pubic area.

With very few exceptions, the men at that Docklands party had waxed or shaved chests, stomachs, pubic, scrotal and anal areas, retaining only armpit hair as a secondary sexual characteristic. The man who had so resented being interrupted as he fucked an epileptic had shaped the central strip into an exclamation mark, with the dot immediately above the root of his penis. Aside from a couple of older men with sparse hair on their chests and stomachs, he was the most hirsute creature there.

I resolved, then, that I too must become a fashion-victim. I started merely with an attempt to tidy up, but found symmetry impossible to maintain. Gradually, as I tried to even things up, the razor encroached first on one side and then the other. At length, I con-cluded that I must remove the lot. Each morning from that day forth I must scrape at what once seemed a modest area of flesh, but now I know to be an extensive acreage on every stretch of which hair seems to grow in a different direction.

It is a long-term commitment. Once stop and there are three weeks of anti-social discomfort to endure before there is a decent, soft, yielding growth. Occasionally I moan about this. I have yet to receive sympathy on this count from a woman.

• • •

I had learned too that there was nothing to fear in swinging. Swingers, in common with most subcultures, welcome new adherents to their cause or calling, and the choice to participate or not is at every point a free one – insofar as any man or woman is free within a few yards of wide eyes or thighs.

Swingers are not predatory. In fact, predators are shunned and despised. And sex – though central to swinging as dancing is to discos or night-clubs – is not its be-all and end-all.

The classic image of an orgy is of wall-to-wall, non-stop sex. This reflects the idleness of film-directors, authors, audiences and readers.

There was certainly ecstatic, cathartic abandon at those parties. There were hours where the entire world seemed made up of warm, firm flesh, damp hair and slippery hot lips and tongues, but even in amongst that enravelment of limbs, there were always jokes and conversations, flirtations and exchanges of gossip and chat.

And the orgy existed in the other rooms where everyone was clothed, because the conversation was as unguarded and uninhibited as the caresses next door, and sex was no longer a threat or a withheld promise. It was an acknowledged, shared means of communication and source of joy.

It is as though swingers are all, say, fighter pilots gathered in the bar, all knowing the wild joys and the dangers of speed and fight, so with no reason to boast of it or to shy from the subject. Swingers who walk in dishevelled and half-clothed – or even naked – after playing, will simply slip into commonplace conversations, debates and games. Appreciative comments or caresses are just that – appreciative, not intrusive or demanding.

Lisa and I were later to introduce Marcus and Nicki – both Oxbridge-educated, good-looking, well-dressed, well-connected and the parents of three – to the Lifestyle. It might be thought that such socially adept people would be the last to complain of inarticulacy.

Both are indeed fluent and apparently at ease in all *milieux*, but Marcus told me, 'I suddenly realised I'd actually been hobbled all my life. Ever since I was very young, I have loved to be with small children and old people, because with them I could have uncomplicated flirtations. I could be open and silly and let random thoughts fly around. I could be unconstrained. I could be me.

'My sexuality – a huge part of who I am – is only allowed to express itself with people who are obviously unavailable by reason of age, or in the process of seduction. Otherwise, I have to mind my words and deaden my eyes and am strictly forbidden to use my body to reach people.'

'Not to mention the neo-Puritans with their new sins,' put in Nicki. 'You should be allowed to say, "Nice arse!" or "God, you're gorgeous" to someone without being arraigned for gross sexism, or shake your booty without being drunk, or show off some fancy new underwear you've bought and are proud of without risking rape ...'

'The great thing about the Lifestyle is that you can flirt openly, you can be yourself, you can use all of your communicative skills without fear,' says Marcus. 'It's a much abused word, but we both feel so liberated, so happy, so natural, as soon as we are amongst players.'

There are many people who attend orgies but – whether because of their own moods or because they encounter no one they fancy – remain clothed throughout and still consider the evening well-spent.

Many women having their menstrual periods will attend parties just for the society. At the end of the evening, there are all the usual rituals of kissing, good-wishes, exchanges of personal information, offers of lifts and the like. This is merely a drinks party that acknowledges its purpose and returns the focus from the drinks to the promotion of closeness between the guests.

On that night I discovered that it was this – the sense of freedom and acceptance, the restoration of natural pride regardless of achievement or accomplishment – which appealed to me about swinging, quite as much as the multifarious sensual pleasures and sexual experiences which it afforded.

Oh, and I learned that the counter-culture mindset can be dangerously pervasive. It is like groping your way from the cinema after watching a movie about a blind person. On the train back to the West Country, I spotted a very attractive blonde woman walking along the corridor towards me. Her faded jeans slicked her long legs like liquid. They made an asterisk at her crotch which winked at me with each step, and she was one of those women who walk with pride in their sexual organs, rather than crouching over them.

She caught my eye. She gave a little smile. Maybe she was on the lookout for sexual diversion. More probably she was merely daydreaming and wondering who I might be that I was looking at her with such undisguised admiration.

I plead in mitigation that I was tired after the previous night's exertions.

She drew nearer.

I reached out to her.

Suddenly Lisa snatched my hand and forced it into my lap. 'No, no no!' she whispered, after the woman had passed. 'Behave yourself! You are back in Don't-Touch-Till-You-Buy Land!'

I sighed. I very much wished that I wasn't.

10

AFTER THE BALL ...

WE MADE FRIENDS ON THAT NIGHT. We received an invitation
to join the Isle of Wight couple on their next visit to their boat. That
was fun. We met more swingers and received further invitations.

My nurse friend was called Gloria. We exchanged telephone numbers and email addresses. She rang a week after the party to ask Lisa
and me to a small dinner party with three other couples at her Laven-
der Hill flat. We accepted.

She and her boyfriend James – a singularly dashing, tall restaura-
teur with an abundance of curly hair – had imposed rules. After the
gnocchi in *brodo*, guests were permitted to kiss one another's lips and
to use only hands in communicating with their neighbours. The
women then changed places. After the *paupiettes* of sole, there was a
twenty-minute break during which the females clambered onto the
table and their male neighbours fed on them, then the women
descended beneath the tablecloth and returned the favour.

Again the women changed places. After the *crème-brulee* with
caramelised fruit and passionfruit sorbet, the table was cleared while

everyone changed into underwear, and only when the women were laid out on the table to their own satisfaction were the men allowed back into the dining-room.

After some diversion there, the whole party adjourned to the living-room, where coffee and a fire were waiting, and played until after four o'clock in the morning.

Sound perhaps best indicates the mood – or moods – of such sessions. At times there are no sounds save the gasps and whimpers of sex, the whisper of fabric, the hushing of skin and the succulent sounds of moist flesh and membrane probing, clutching, releasing and reclaiming. At times there is desultory chat, or there are jokes flung around. At times fucking becomes fierce in one section of the room, and the women take peculiar pleasure and laugh deep and affectionate as they study the faces and hear the obscenities and squeals of their fellows.

Eventually the air is filled with the percussion of flesh slapping flesh, with male grunts and growls and, above all, with rhythmic female glottal stops – some attached to yelps, some to sighs, some to quizzical whimpers, some to rising keenings, some standing alone, staccato, sequential and mounting to fierce, gravelly roars.

We were also invited to accompany other couples on visits to paid-entry private house parties and clubs. After the first few such evenings, I realised that that Coupleszone party – although small and civilised – had been very basic in terms of facilities. Most other private parties offer at least a dance floor, a hot-tub or two, a swimming pool in summer, a dark room for the more modest or indiscriminate, and at least one sex-swing in one or other of the playrooms.

In common with many an inhibited Western male, I tend to avoid dance floors. I can just about waltz, enjoy jiving (though less so since I gave up alcohol, and I suspect the women of England may be grateful for my sobriety) and can manage a cramped night-club shuffle, which is, after all, merely an inhibited perpendicular orgy.

Dance floors at real orgies, however, are particularly erotic. In our culture dancing has become a predominantly female form of self-expression, and here women can dance erotically with one another rather than with handbags. A great deal of kissing takes place. Clothes are rucked or flap loose as they circle one another, rub up against one another or nuzzle into one another's concavities. This is the other sort of play, as old as that which takes place in the playrooms.

I quickly learned to avoid dark rooms. Many a shy novice (and yes, there are shy orgiasts) tends to head first for these havens. Most experienced players, however, prefer to see with whom they are playing.

Some people have better reasons than mere modesty for wishing to hide their faces and bodies, and – in the darkness and the tangle of limbs – believe they are free to paw every body that comes within reach. Of course, if they persist, they will be removed and will not be allowed to return, but it can be unpleasant to emerge into the light to realise which monsters have been mauling you.

Most parties also boast a private room or two. Here coy couples and their friends resort for private or semi-private play – a convention which I simply could not understand. Why attend a swingers' party only to seek privacy once there?

The rule here is simple. If the door is closed, it must remain closed, and intruders are unwelcome. If it is left open or ajar, spectators are welcome and can approach those already playing to ask if they can join them. A hopeful caress is not suitable here. The fact that the incumbents have resorted to a private room, rather than an open playroom, means that only an explicit request is acceptable.

Many 'vanillas' claim that they would like to try swinging but dread the notion of meeting colleagues or acquaintances from another section of their lives – neighbours, the bank manager or their children's teachers – at a party or through a swingers' meet.

Some swingers naively insist that they will not play within a fifty-mile radius of their own homes. They inevitably bump into others who think the same and who tend to be the very people whom they want to avoid.

Haphazard meetings do occur. I have met old schoolfriends, my GP and her boyfriend, former colleagues and neighbours at swing parties.

But what of it? We all know why we are there, just as we would know if we met at a restaurant that we were both there to perform the similarly 'bestial' process of eating. Did we assume before such a meeting that these people did not have sex lives, that they had no genitals, or that their children were immaculately conceived? And they are there for the same reasons.

It is also not uncommon to encounter faces and bodies familiar from television, or from newspaper byline mugshots, amidst the melee. Again, what of it? They are neither breaking the law nor abusing the unwilling. They are there to have fun. Save in the case of a swinging journalist or TV presenter who is morally censorious or sexually illiberal in his or her public pronouncements, there is no public interest defence for breaching their privacy or that of private clubs or parties.

On the two occasions when I have witnessed disturbances at parties, the police have been called without hesitation and have behaved with good-humoured respect on their arrival.

They would be ill-advised to do otherwise. A police raid on the average swing party would result in the arrests of several naked police officers, solicitors and barristers of both genders, and – until the intrusive, 'nanny-state' EU so far violates constitutional British liberties as to proscribe sexual activities between adults – any resulting prosecution would be sneered out of court.

One woman whom I met at a private party admitted that it had been 'a bit of a shock' to look up from a pile of writhing bodies 'with my mouth full of pussy and some guy fucking me from behind' to find her widowed and long-estranged father, stark naked and rampant, looking down on her.

After the initial shock, the experience brought them closer together. 'So much for language. I thought we had nothing in common. Now we can compare notes and have a giggle, though we do ring one another to check what parties we are attending so we avoid any more unpleasant surprises.'

This is another excellent reason for avoiding the dark rooms at parties.

11

SWING-CLUBS

WITHIN SIX WEEKS, WE HAD visited three swing-clubs – Chameleons (my all-time favourite) in Darlaston, Birmingham; Swingers' Junction at Totton in the New Forest; and AbFab near Staines and Heathrow Airport.

Swingers' clubs are run along the same principles as private parties. They can be expected to have social rooms and playrooms, darkrooms, hot-tubs, saunas, sex-swings, usually dance floors and occasionally cinemas, which show pornographic movies but in effect are merely dark rooms which afford players the opportunity to play in nostalgic circumstances. Some have steam rooms, dungeons and other themed rooms. Some have swimming pools – indoors or outdoors.

Even more than with private parties, which tend to be consistent in their requirements, it is necessary to check what sort of night is on offer before attending a club. Those seeking a gentle 'couples and single girls only' evening do not wish to turn up on one of the nights when selected single males are admitted, or a 'Greedy Girls' night where there is an abundance of single males, many of them unversed in swinging decorum and only incidentally interested in social inter-action.

It is also worth double-checking membership criteria (for single females and for couples, this is usually a formality at the door) and licensing. An increasing number of clubs are licensed to sell alcohol, but some can sell only soft drinks and require guests to bring their own wine or beer.

Orgies make even the most fastidious eaters hungry. All clubs and parties therefore supply at least a supermarket bog-standard buffet. It is hardly worth pointing out that any meals taken before setting off to play should be small, nourishing and light. Fish, bananas (many women swear that they make men's semen taste better, and the potassium and carbohydrate can do no harm), parsley, pineapple and smoothies are highly recommended.

Dutch courage, however, beyond a few glasses of wine on arrival, is not. Drink is taken sparingly at parties. Swingers like to remember their adventures. These are glamorous and fantastic enough to require no soft-focus.

From that first party it took six weeks to feel entirely at home in the swinging *milieu*, to have invitations and friendly messages con-stantly flowing into our inbox, to have feedback on the principal websites, and to know the language, the protocol and our likes and dislikes.

And I had thought that, without alcohol, I would never again readily fit into any social set aside from Alcoholics Anonymous.

● ● ●

My advice to others entering this world for the first time is simple. They should behave as if they were at any other party – circulate rather than remaining with one obviously congenial couple or group, consider the feelings of others, particularly those less confident than you, and assist your hosts and hostesses. Do not hasten to play. Enjoy the party regardless of the playrooms.

Courtesy need not wait for its reward in heaven. The couple that has made friends and conveyed confidence to others will soon be able to count on acceptance – easily the most important property in a sub-culture where strangers are welcome but regarded with caution.

On the other hand, be sure after a couple of hours to retire to a playroom and play together. Not only is this helpful to hosts by supplying a valuable lead to many guests who may be more hesitant than you, but it establishes beyond doubt that you are of the fraternity.

It frequently happens, too, that the playrooms very suddenly fill up and, when you look for a space in which to join the fun, you find that the only empty spaces are flanked by couples with whom you would sooner not be naked, let alone run the risk that they might seek to play with you.

For all that the Lifestyle is quite properly inclusive of all shapes and ages, neither I nor any of my regular swing partners find grossly fat people appealing, believing – as a general rule – that those who cannot, or will not, look after their own bodies are unlikely to look after ours very well either. It is very frustrating to stand in a doorway, eager to play, only to find that you have to squeeze in between lately erupted – but barely congealed – human volcanoes.

Stake a claim instead to a corner of a selected playroom and, when attractive people met previously appear in the doorway, indicate with smiles that they are welcome. With luck, Congenial Corner will become established and grow, allowing you to take a break for a drink or a cigarette and return to find friends, or friends of friends, still playing there.

PART IV

1

DEFINING TERMS

IN MY NEW-FOUND ENTHUSIASM and elation, I realised that I would have to defend and explain swinging to critical friends. They all seemed to have clear ideas as to what the word meant – it was 'wife-swapping', it was 'polyamory', it was 'orgies'. In one instance (clearly someone who had read and trusted too many Sunday newspapers), it was 'squalid suburban sex games. And stuff.'

The more I examined it, however, the more I struggled for an accurate definition.

At first sight, it all seems so clear. Swinging, widely known as 'the Lifestyle', is recreational sex – or the social life which includes and accepts recreational sex – between two or more people who meet with the explicit purpose of enjoying sexual activity together, generally without further commitment or emotional involvement.

It often entails the swapping or sharing of conventional partners or spouses. It often entails attendance at parties or orgies, where those attending may have several sexual encounters with several people in one afternoon, evening or night.

And yet, whilst all of this is true, none of it is constantly true

enough to rank as a definition. The statement is peppered with qual-
ifying adverbs – 'generally', 'frequently' and so on.

Non-swingers who attend nightclubs or discos, after all, often do
so with the purpose of finding partners for recreational sex, however
much they may pretend that they are looking for love or friendship.

Neither love nor friendship is particularly well served by the short
skirt, the sliver of fabric barely concealing the breasts, the cock-of-
the-roost strut or the gut-wriggle and bump-and-grind thrust of the
pubis on the dance floor. All these are the semaphore of oestrus,
whether or not one or both parties impose restraints before intercourse.

'Generally without further commitment or emotional involvement' ... Well, yes. That is the intention, as it is the intention of
many who have 'casual' sex or engage prostitutes, but in all these
instances I know of profounder attachments made in the course of
such encounters.

Swingers may like sex with strangers, but they also like to make
friends with those strangers and to feel at ease with them. They are,
after all, kindred spirits who share a hobby and an attitude not
merely to sexuality, but to life and libertarianism in general.

'I'm a member of the MG Owner's Club,' said Tara, a 41-year-old
housewife and boutique manager whom I met at a club in Sheffield.
'Does that mean I'm obsessed with cars? Aside from saying, "Hey!
Nice car!" when we see one in the car park, we never really talk cars
at our meetings, and I wouldn't know a carburettor from a big end.
We're just people linked by an interest and a sort of general attitude,
so we meet, have a few drinks and make friends. It's the same with
swinging.'

Other swingers have made similar comparisons between swinging
and football supporters' clubs, swinging and AA ... There are even
subcultures within the swinging subculture – 'Swingers on Bikes',
'Swingers in Caravans' and the like.

Inevitably, in any such *milieu*, protectiveness and particular affections will spring up.

As to 'sharing' and 'swapping' partners, this implies an ownership alien to the Lifestyle.

If you cannot own or sell a human being, how can you swap or share one? Yes, swingers tend – when in couples – to encourage and to smile upon and, where desirable, to participate in their partners' enjoyment of others. But even this is not invariably true.

Many so-called swinging couples search – largely in vain – for another female for their mutual pleasure or merely for that of the women, excluding any male participation. Many others will seek out single men but rule out the involvement of other females. And again, many will attend swing-clubs for the view and the companionship, but will only have sex with one another. A significant section of the Lifestyle consists of couples who never play with others, but merely enjoy the ease and the liberty afforded by the ambience and the company.

So-called 'soft swingers' engage in oral sex, intimate caressing and kissing with others, but regard penetrative sex as their own exclusive terrain, and advertise themselves as 'ultimate own partner only'. We who are listed on SDC.com as 'full swap' sometimes lay bets on how long they will maintain this lofty principle. It is usually the female who first breaks and, after the first few months of playing, asks that the restriction be set aside. But some couples remain resolutely 'soft swap' for decades.

All these call themselves 'swingers'.

As for orgies, many swingers do not attend these at all, preferring to chat on the net and the telephone for weeks, months or even years before meeting their chosen playmates, and even then insisting upon lengthy drinks and dinners before they consent to engage in physical intimacy. Yet still these call themselves 'swingers'.

Most swingers play freely in, and in front of, crowds, yet some *soi disant* swingers are so reluctant to perform sexually in front of others, including even their own partners, that they insist on 'separate room' sex – a strange ritual far closer to the wife-swapping of yore.

And, of course, many 'vanillas' have experience of threesomes and exhibitionist sex in larger groups, but do not call themselves, nor think of themselves as, 'swingers'.

Swinging is broadly divided into private 'meets' and parties. The private meets – usually organised after a brief exchange on the Internet and a few telephone calls – are where one couple, single man or single woman will visit another and, if the chemistry is there, have sex and perhaps make friends. At parties it is the same process, but this is obviously hastened amidst a crowd.

Briefly, the party has the advantages that there is no embarrassing prelude (the shuffling of feet, the glancing at watches, the set of signals whereby members of a couple indicate to each other that each finds both members of the other couple attractive or otherwise) or aftermath (the showing to the guest room afterwards, the breakfast with the family). And there is a larger selection of potential playmates from whom to choose, as well as the stimulus of group sex all around you.

The meet is preferred by some precisely because it is more intimate, and because the degree of exhibitionism required of the party-goer is not common to all players.

In fact, the only term which may lay claim to being constantly true in my previous attempt at definition is 'explicit'. Swingers' purposes are explicit. They openly state that they are seeking partners for sex.

So, of course, are many people at drinks parties, clubs and bars, but they attempt to disguise the fact. Swingers organise their sex lives where others allow a greater degree of the haphazard and the opportunist to ordain them.

As part of that organisation, swingers have strict rules which are transgressed only with explicit and exceptional sanction. Paramount amongst these are 'No means no' and 'Safe sex will at all times be practised'.

And that, really, seems to be that. Swingers are very, very diverse, and it is only that explicit acknowledgement of their ends, that blanket acceptance of the rules, which marks them out from 'vanillas' or non-swingers.

2

SUBCATEGORIES

ALMOST EVERY OTHER ATTEMPT at a definition of swinging links it to the fetish scene. There are many connections and crossover points, but in fact those links are tenuous.

I use the term 'fetish' here to mean not just bondage and sado-masochism (BDSM), peculiar anatomical fixations and all the associated apparel and apparatus, but more specifically an avowed, constant and general sexual preference. Even Krafft Ebing acknowledged that fetishism – 'I adore my partner's breasts/toes/knickers, etc' – is a feature of the most conventional monogamous pairings.

So, yes, female swingers own towering heels, thigh-high boots, corsets, whips, restraints, PVC, leather corsets and the like. These are, after all, standard props of sexual role-play, and most swingers' clubs have a 'dungeon' equipped with paddles, leg and wrist restraints and the like. Equally, many a 'fetishist' swings – that is, seeks out and sometimes has sex with partners who share his or her predilection.

The longer I have been on the scene, however, the more the divide between the two groups seems to gape.

Of course swingers dress up in fetish gear and play bondage games. So do most of us without any such subculture status, just as most ordinary lovers play role-play and spanking games.

Fetishists, however, are by definition sexually aroused by their specific activities and the objects related to them more than – or rather than – the people with whom they perform them. The word 'fetish' generally indicates an icon or a practice which displaces more familiar lusts or adherences and becomes an end in itself. It is the idolatry of sexuality.

The fetish parties that we have attended are great fun and very, very picturesque. They are playful, as are swing-parties, but tend to involve surprisingly little sex and a great deal of prinking, preening and admiring frottage.

Costumes, role play and narcissism are at their heart rather than the hot and sticky activities at swinging's centre. Fetishists dress up for their pleasures, where swingers find liberation and joy in undressing and celebrating common frailties.

I expect a chorus of protest from swingers who enjoy the 'fet' scene and fetishists who regularly swing. I maintain nonetheless that, whilst swinging is all about close contact, nakedness and commonalty, fetishism – or the scene which claims that name – is principally concerned with illusion, individuality and otherness.

For all that, there are fetishists who are swingers, just as there are members of just about every other social and sexual subcategory.

Just to list a few, there are men – usually, but not always, older than their partners – who rarely have sex themselves but enjoy watching their partners doing so and look to provide them with pleasures which they no longer seek or feel.

My partners and I have, I think, played with people of just about every race save the Inuit. But whenever we encounter a delicious Filipina or Thai girl at a party, we always look around for her older, portlier and often inactive partner. We also tend – often very reluctantly

– to avoid her, because we can seldom be sure, for all her enthusiastic smiles and giggles, that she is a free and entirely willing participant.

There are also, however, men who specifically seek the pleasures of frustration and humiliation caused by their own inactivity, whilst their female partners indulge lavish fantasies in front of them. These we will happily indulge.

Then there are voyeurs of both genders who seldom if ever join in but take their pleasure simply in the associated social life and in watching what is, after all, the cheapest and best live porn show (or *tableau vivant*) that they will ever know.

There are occasional callow young men who rent or cajole a woman (known as 'a ticket') into swinging and then expect to have free rein with others present. These do not last long. Their intentions are too urgent, too immediate, their actions too intrusive to be anything less than obvious, and the women recruited for such purposes inevitably give the game away, either accidentally through disinterest or deliberately through solidarity with other swinging women. Such people, when recognised, are ejected.

There are a few women who attend parties with the explicit intention of being gang-banged or fulfilling some other fantasy (I know two who went through a phase of attending parties blindfold). Often these are one-off adventures. Sometimes – rarely – they will become regular diversions.

3

BISEXUALITY IN SWINGING

ONE OF THE SADDEST AND SILLIEST legacies of Victorian repression and Freudianism is the association of individuals with really quite ridiculously broad but specific 'sexualities' – the insistence that a man or woman is essentially 'homosexual' or 'heterosexual', 'sadistic', 'masochistic' or whatever.

Needless to say, the activities associated with these labels have been practised throughout human history. Ancient Greeks and Romans, mediaeval and Renaissance men and women – all have acknowledged and enjoyed sexual desires for their own genders and divers games, generally without incurring excessive social displeasure or ostracism.

Certainly none would have understood the notion of classification simply on the basis of these activities or preferences. The words 'homosexual' and 'heterosexual' did not even exist until 1862, and Krafft Ebing coined 'sadism' and 'masochism' only in 1886.

After years of observing swingers, and particularly the way in which women behave when freed to seek pleasure where and how they will, I believe more than ever that such terminology is mistaken and misleading.

There is plenty of bisexual activity in swinging and, of course, the swing-scene allows players to explore this part of their natures without strictures, commitment or the perils of possessiveness.

Women seem especially pragmatic about this, as about most things. At least 80 per cent of all swinging women with whom I have played, or whom I have interviewed regularly, have sexual contact with other women. This is not to say that it is obligatory or that exclusively 'straight' women are made to feel alien.

'I don't think it's the same for men in our society,' says Lisa. 'It seems to demand a whole change of mindset for them to enjoy one another's bodies. I guess it's because of that aggressive, intrusive organ and all that conditioning which tells them that another man's body is of its nature dirty or a threat, and that sex always means invasion and ejaculation. So there's more fight-or-flight adrenaline triggered than sexual juices.

'For me, it's just natural and logical. Take all the sacred commitment stuff from sex, and a woman's body is just a warm, lovely, responsive, exciting source of pleasure, very different from a man, but oh, so delicious and absorbing.'

Katy, a 24-year-old former naval rating who was to become my swing partner for a year, also recognises that swinging enables her to enjoy pleasures which otherwise she denies herself for practical reasons. 'I love to have sex with women, and to feel and taste their excitement. I can really get totally lost in there. It's like the most total ecstatic focus I know ... I suppose I've had sex with a good half of my best and closest girlfriends, but if I do that out there in the vanilla world, I have them hanging around making demands on me, and playing mind-reading games, and being jealous and all that stuff. Swinging, I can play with them, love them and adore all that very special sensuality without all that shit, and it's great.'

Male bisexuality is widespread on the one-to-one meet scene, where advertisers will clearly state themselves to be 'bi' or 'bi-curious'. It is far rarer on the party scene, or, at least, far less obvious, not least because many swingers of both genders still find male gay sex a turn-off and, in truth, because many 'homosexual' men in our society also find heterosexual sex if not distasteful, at least unconducive.

I believe this to be a generational thing. I know many younger swingers who find it a turn-on. Some female swingers resent the absence of male bisexual activity. 'The men get to see us getting it on all the time,' complains Natalia, 26, a beautiful Siberian swinger married to a Somerset businessman. 'I always hope to see men together, but it doesn't happen much. It's not fair.'

Several older women to whom I have spoken, however, maintain (such is the prevalence, even here, of nineteenth-century bipolar classifications) that, 'If a man says he's bi, he's actually gay.'

Those men who have accepted labelling as 'homosexual' therefore tend, like women who believe themselves lesbians, to have their own contact networks, websites and clubs.

For all that, male homosexual activity (usually restricted to caressing and oral, and only with explicit consent) is not unknown in the melee of an orgy. The true homophobic is well advised to stay away – not least because swingers – in Europe at least – feel a profound affinity with 'gay' men, who, like them, have for so long been marginalised for a lifestyle choice or propensity which harms, and so should concern, no-one.

4

BONOBOSEXUALITY

ONE WAY OR ANOTHER, I seem to be further than ever from a clear and concise definition of the swinging hobby.

Try again, then. It is social activity that freely admits of (but does not require) sex which, if it happens, is smiled upon and approved by the partners of those engaged. It is largely an activity of the otherwise monogamous and law-abiding.

Above all, and as distinct from almost every other sexual playground in our society, swinging is wholly conducted according to the requirements of females, who ordain the ambience, the style and the pace of swingers' events, and of each sexual or social encounter.

Sometimes, despairing of explaining to vanillas why swingers enjoy their hobby, I shrug and resort to, 'Well, maybe we just have more bonobo genes where you are all chimp.'

Bonobos are – with chimpanzees – our closest relatives in the animal world. Whereas theoretically monogamous chimpanzees spend their lives in screeching and squabbling and frequently murdering one another, bonobos are matriarchal, pensive, socially cooperative and peaceable, and engage in routine recreational sex, regardless of fertility (indeed including a great deal of oral and female on female sex) as a means of greeting, bonding, peacemaking and simply as a leisure activity.

Will the moralist then declare the chimp superior to, or 'better than', the bonobo?

'Bonobos have sex most of the time ... a fairly quick, perfunctory, and relaxed activity that functions as a social cement,' writes Tim Taylor, of Bradford University. 'But for cultural constraints, we would all behave more like bonobos. In physical terms, there is actually nothing that bonobos do that some humans do not sometimes do.'

And maybe, after all, my glib explanation has some foundation in fact. Could there be strings of genetic information common to bonobos in swingers, but missing in the DNA of our disapproving chimp brethren?

Maybe swingers and their kind warrant a new sexual subdivision, a category which spans homosexual and heterosexual preferences and is far more consistently distinctive than either of these – bonobosexuals, born into a chimp-dominated society.

There is no point in proselytising. Chimps will – and no doubt should – remain chimps. Their bonobo cousins, however, also need to be themselves but not to damage others or the valuable social structures which preserve them. Like human 'gays', they largely accept the chimp way of life and try not to force their activities on them, but simply recognise that it is not, in every regard, for them.

It is just rather sad that chimp-humans do not display the same tolerance and understanding towards their close kin.

5

IN DEFENCE OF HEDONISM

THE CURIOUS THING ABOUT the above attempt at a definition is that it seems to identify swingers as more, not less, civilised and courteous than their vanilla confreres.

Swingers insist upon rules and mutuality in the fulfilment of their lusts. They reject deceit and moral and emotional ambiguity. They look to create fantastic, amusing and luxurious environments for their pleasures.

It is surely a characteristic mark of civilisation that we hang our paintings in gilt frames and prefer to see them in beautiful and tranquil surroundings, that we clothe ourselves in fine, tailored fabrics rather than in roughly stitched skins and that we prepare our food with artifice and devote enormous effort to the costume, décor and ambient sounds in which it is enjoyed.

How is it, then, that the man – which is to say almost every man – who climbs a murky stairwell to avail himself of a prostitute, or the woman – which is to say almost every woman – who kindly but grudgingly yields to 'amorous' advances for the sake of domestic peace, may be regarded as morally and socially respectable, whilst the swinger is a morally irresponsible savage?

It was initially hard for me to get my head around the notion that hedonism is by definition morally responsible.

The Romans and their Christian successors may have claimed the respectable name of hedonism for their revels, but, except perhaps for the common crowd at their Mayday and Christmas festivals, these were no more hedonistic than the adolescent's guilt-ridden, resentful, tortuous, solitary indulgences or the unconvinced atheist's graffito 'Sod God'. They were rebellious, iconoclastic, exploitative and frequently brutish.

Today's binge-drinkers also claim hedonism as their justification, but they too seek to silence intellect in riotous disorder rather than to harmonise their faculties. As a specialist in both, I can confidently assert that having enthusiasts getting off on one's face is infinitely more ecstatic than getting off it solo by means of booze.

Of course orgies have a long history as religious observances. Women with little mirrors on their dresses therefore often ask whether the orgiastic experience is 'spiritual'. This is a characteristically Christian question which presupposes a distinction – even a contradistinction – between the spiritual and the physical.

Hedonism bids to integrate body, soul and intellect, 'animal', human and divine. It does not seek, as do most doctrinaire modern religions and the consciously vicious reactions to them, to assert one by denying the other.

Christianity assumes that sex is evil at once because it is pleasurable and because it is developed from a primitive, animalistic and ultimately irresistible imperative. Sex is acknowledged and permitted only insofar as it is quite evidently necessary (even the most psychotic zealot must accept that his parents did it at least once) or, with hubristic impudence, 'sanctioned' by man-made law. Self-hatred – despite of 'the flesh' – is an inherent component of Christian doctrine.

Monotheism itself dissociates the Creator from His creation and asserts the existence of an idealised spirit-world distinct from the physical. If God inhabits the one, the other must perforce be inferior and hostile.

This notion is fostered by the Judaeo-Christian Creation myth – surely the first semi-autobiographical novel and a psychopathological case study at that. Adam and Eve were childlike but happy. They attained sexual maturity and so fell from grace. Their shame has been visited upon subsequent generations to this day.

The cruciform nature of history with Christ at its groin also helps the moralists. To this day, willy nilly, we see world history as thus divided, with nature-worship and primitivism at one open end of the cross and 'civilisation', 'progress' and monogamy at the other, for all that the latter 'V' is a paltry two millennia in length and progress appears wholly illusory. This is a patent nonsense, but a powerful one for all that.

With such dissociation at the core of our culture, happiness is rarely if ever unalloyed. Joy in your own body and senses, or in those of another, is habitually tempered by guilt and a sense of dirtiness and inadequacy. Genital stirrings are culpable. A clear distinction is insisted upon between erotica and art, physical and spiritual.

Enjoyment of music, landscape, weather or animals for example is invariably ascribed to freedom from other lusts or hungers. It is detached – 'spiritual', by which is generally meant auditory, visual and cerebral, as distinct from senses more visceral and less pre-dictable in the responses which they may trigger. So 'beautiful views' of nature are best seen through car windows or the bars of a zoo, sani-tised and rendered safe by distance.

The hunter, the artist and the hedonist constitute a class apart. All seek out and assert the interdependence and essential unity of all beings by enjoying and celebrating creation. All are intensely physi-cal. All seek to negate the intrusive, judgemental self rather than aspiring to some distorted, idealistic illusion of how humans and the earth might be.

The hunter, who must sink into his environment and become very small; the painter, who asserts rather than disguises the earthy muckiness of paint in rendering inner reality; the poet to whom abstract nouns and ideals are by definition anaethema; the lover, who worships at the ultimate shrines of human mortality; the gourmet, who seeks only the innermost truth and nature of ingredients and their interrelations (I am tempted to add 'the mother', for whom love is frequently burdensome, irritating, messy, compulsory and without illusion) – all reject perfectibilism and idealism. All worship the universal through the particular, the 'creator' through creation. All get their hands dirty.

To none of these, surely, does the question 'Is it spiritual?' make the slightest sense.

How can there be spiritual joy without physical fitness, and, by the same token, how can physical pleasure exist without spiritual contentment? How can integral pleasure exist in the awareness of pain, exploitation, coercion or injustice? These must mar the apprehension of pleasure or beauty, and assert the presence of the perceiver as an alien intruder.

The irresponsibility and freedom from external concerns sought by the hedonist is therefore wholly dependent on moral responsibility. Our fellow participants must be willing and happy. We must be satisfied that our actions will not leave emotional or physical debris.

Pleasure in sex is seldom dissociated in everyday life from long-term emotional expectations, proprietorial trespass, deceit or tedious and burdensome responsibilities. Sex is at best naughty, at worst sinful, and the voice of conscience is best ignored by drowning it out with alcohol, drugs and angry excess – a long, long way from innocent play or from 'ecstasy', whose literal meaning is 'standing outside oneself' or 'getting out of it.'

So the rebellious erotomane attacks himself and the erotic within him. The hedonist, however, seeks to combine stimuli – music, food, costume, textures, scents, sounds, sights, sensations – to banish obtruding causes for distaste or worries (ecstasy fuelled by McDonald's or Madonna must surely be impossible). That means that moral doubts or fears must also be excluded. Hedonism, in denying moral responsibility, presupposes it as a prerequisite.

Anyhow, swingers can find spiritual authority if we really seek it. It comes from the altogether more harmonious, less humanocentric precepts of Taoism. 'If a man continually changes the women with whom he has intercourse, the benefit will be great,' says Yu-fang-pi-chueh in *I-shin-po*. 'If in one night he can have intercourse with more than ten women it is best ...'

Having tried this path to enlightenment on three successive birthdays – once with a playground roundabout, converted to carry six prone bodies in a very warm and welcoming human asterisk – I can highly recommend it.

6

WHEN THE FUN WAS TAKEN OUT OF SEX

SWINGING IS A MID-TWENTIETH-CENTURY attempt to resolve problems which started – or, at least, were institutionalised – more than a century before. The word 'play' had been widely used for sex until the end of the seventeenth century. It has been fortuitously rediscovered by swingers today.

Until 1800 or thereabouts, there were innumerable forms of sexual play – shared caresses, kisses, oral and interfemoral intercourse, mutual masturbation, coitus (if at all) interruptus – and female orgasm was considered as essential as male. It was believed that male and female each contributed a necessary seed in orgasmic ejaculation.

It has always surprised me that modern feminists (unlike Germaine Greer) accept the word 'vagina', the Latin for 'sheath', which casts that organ as an appendage dependent for its function upon the male. This is a modern concept. Until the 1680s, the correct term was 'neck of the womb'. It was an organ in its own right, not dependent upon a penis or a child for its function.

In the eighteenth century, with the recognition of sexes as 'separate' (though all subsequent discoveries have tended to support the earlier concept of modified androgynes), and of semen as the precipitating agent in conception, sex came exclusively to mean penetrative intercourse culminating in male ejaculation. The neck of the womb ceased to have an autonomous existence.

By 1800, what had been 'play' and a pleasurable end in itself had become mere 'foreplay' and the pussy just a furrow in which to sow.

The consequences were truly dire. If sex was invariably likely to impregnate, it followed that it was dangerous and should at every turn be restricted to the committed. Sex and romantic love became inextricably, if improbably, linked. Fucking guaranteed male orgasm but did little for the prospects of female, which became a matter of minor importance and ultimately of shame. Mutuality and equality in other regards also went by the board.

Conceptions outside marriage rocketed. Masturbation of all varieties was classified as a grave sin and, ultimately, as a mortal sickness.

Paradoxically too, pornography enjoyed its first golden age, and imposed its own phallocentric logic upon Western sexuality. Play – heterosexual and homosexual – is interminable, its dynamic diffuse. Literary form, however, demands a start and a more or less inexorable progress towards an end. Just as fiction requires marriage or death as a convenient culmination, so pornography (in eighteenth-century literature no less than modern film) found its necessary apotheosis in male ejaculation.

The clitoris meanwhile became an irrelevant 'little' appendage rather than the tip of an internal system larger than the penis and requiring more blood when fully engorged. Within a few decades, it had sunk beneath the waves of ignorance, and the few brave Western men who sought it did so with all the trepidation, uncertainty and gallantry of Burton and Speke as they plunged into the interior in search of the source of the Nile. Freud famously perpetuated the notion of the clitoris as a 'stunted penis'.

Homosexuality in consequence of this new concept meant sodomy, whilst female homosexuality became simply meaningless. You could not have sex without penetration. Jealousy and moral outrage at extra-marital sexual adventures were justified.

In the eighteenth century, the fun was taken out of sex.

The one childlike, carefree, fantasy escape from day-to-day responsibility, worry and posturing, became – preposterously – a serious 'adult' business. Paradoxically, adults also considered it beneath their dignity and infantile, yet strictly proscribed any mention of it in the presence of children,

This was surely wicked enough in itself, but when the fun, mutuality and constant negotiability of pleasure in sexual play vanished, so did all mutuality and negotiability in relations between the genders.

The eighteenth-century obscurantism which condemned all, save phallocentric penetration and ejaculation, and converted women to passive recipients of these – so rendering all sex a lifelong commitment – became formalised in the nineteenth century by means of bad law, bad medicine, bad education and generally bad art. It persisted throughout the Western world way into the twentieth century. We inherited that tragic legacy.

Today with women and men once more enjoying mutuality, and with contraception all but ubiquitous and effective, play has been reintroduced. The clitoris has re-emerged from the depths (though its precise location on the map remains a mystery to many Western men). Oral sex and female bisexuality are probably more widespread and commonly accepted at every level of society than at any time in modern British history.

This time, thanks to cheap and efficient condoms, play commonly includes fucking (as opposed to interfemoral – between the thighs – sex in the seventeenth century), but fucking is neither its purpose nor necessarily its most intimate form of expression.

I believe that contemporary swingers have unwittingly rediscovered sexual play within a structured society, and are at the forefront of a movement which will do more to restore equality between the genders than all the political activism and academic pontificating which has preceded it.

7

THE LIBERATING CONDOM

THE NOTION, MUCH PROPAGATED in the wake of AIDS, that all homosexuals are by nature promiscuous, was and is absurd. As well argue that racial origins predispose a human being to musicality or that (as was frequently asserted) homosexuals were more likely than heterosexuals to be paedophile.

What is true is that many homosexuals, whether in long-term emotional relationships or not, felt freer to engage in sexual acts for shared pleasure and the concomitant joys of companionship than did heterosexual men and women in the late, unlamented age of phallo-centricity.

The associations evoked by (and the real risks entailed in) male ejaculation in the vagina properly inhibited heterosexuals. It brought a real gun into an otherwise enjoyable game of cowboys. It takes more than awareness of a pill wholly to dispel associations with preg-nancy, possession and jealousy.

In this sense, the homosexual denizens of the '70s bath-house were the Baptists of today's swingers (the famous gay Continental Baths in the basement of Manhattan's Ansonia Hotel made way for the heterosexual swingers' club Plato's Retreat). Like swingers, they frequently played as loving, emotionally committed couples, enjoying the intimacy of watching one another at play with others, and sharing one another's pleasures.

The acknowledgement of gay rights was an acknowledgement too of divergent sexual preferences and of sexual play as a companionable pleasure, rather than merely as a sacramental commitment or a process with a specific function. Where laws changed to recognise *equal* rights for gays, they afforded to such pleasure the status of a necessity rather than that of a mere indulgence.

If AIDS checked the homosexual play culture, it paradoxically liberated that of heterosexuals. The sudden routine acceptance of condoms in all penetrative sex – save with one trusted partner – sundered mere sensual pleasure from the proprietorial, proscriptive view of sex which had held the Western world in thrall for two centuries. Play became play again, and distinct from the serious business of procreation.

Swingers are faithful to their spouses and partners. Though they may play with hundreds of others, they do not have illicit affairs or unprotected, private, penetrative sex, save with their own partners. The distinction may appear minimal to those who have no experience of it, but it is a valid one.

I hesitate to parody the old moralistic saw. It is altogether too slick. I yield to temptation only because it genuinely seems to be true: the couple that plays together stays together.

8

THE ORIGINS OF SWINGING

THE HISTORY OF SWINGING – that is, of a recognised, organised milieu explicitly and routinely dedicated to meetings and parties for the purposes of sexual gratification for both genders – is generally held to have begun during or immediately after World War II.

Certainly war has a destabilising effect on social structures and sexual constraints, and this was a very special war. The vastly increased mobility and freedom afforded to women of every class (and the sudden visibility of the pleasures of the already sexually liberal upper-classes), coupled with the unparalleled absence of barriers between genders, created an unprecedented climate for erotic experiment.

Grass widows in past wars had repined in their husbands' absence on active service. In World War II Britain, however, they were surrounded not just by very old and very young males but by young, active, often exotic and similarly frustrated young men stationed or on leave.

Restaurants, pubs and nightclubs enjoyed an unprecedented boom in cities enlivened by the constant awareness of death and danger, not merely at the front but in the nightly Russian roulette of the blitz in the streets and squares of home.

The old provocation to incontinence – the awareness that a young man was about to face death in the trenches and should not die virgin or unappreciated – was no longer experienced just once a war, or once a year, but all but daily. Soldiers and sailors continually enjoyed leave in the fleshpots of home, then returned to active service far away. Fliers commuted daily to battle.

Illicit affairs, often involving parties committed to other long-standing relationships, were commonplace. Many in consequence sought to play. Anal penetration is commonly recorded. Condoms no longer had to be bought from under the counter in barbers' shops. They were distributed in a serviceman's rations. Briefly, sex became explicitly short-term pleasure and companionship rather than a commitment to long-term bondage.

Terry Gould, in his excellent *The Lifestyle: A Look at the Erotic Rites of Swingers* – the only intelligent book to date impartially to record the scene – maintains that it was amongst the most obviously gladiatorial and glamorous of warriors, American fighter pilots, that organised swinging first emerged. Their high fatality rate and their penchant for risk-taking (evidently shared by their wives) caused them to start sharing spouses 'as a kind of tribal bonding ritual, with a tacit understanding that the two-thirds of the husbands who survived would look after the widows.'

Whether or not this last intention was indeed implicit, the circumstances – elite *esprit de corps*, isolation from the wider community, high income, low life-expectancy and long periods of boredom alternating with short, ecstatic periods of high risk – were propitious for such a development.

Organised swinging (as distinct from disorganised adultery which shatters interdependence) does create a strong communal bond, not least because of its secrecy from the clothed, vanilla world.

What is clear is that swinging started in suburban military officers' quarters at some stage between 1945 and 1953, by which time it was well – if sparsely – established in the white-collar population throughout the United States.

No one seems able to establish whether the 'key club' or 'key party' – at which men dropped their keys into a hat and women drew them out at random, so selecting their next sex-partners – ever actually existed. If so, embryonic swinging was as different from its present-day incarnation as a peculiarly ugly duckling from a full-grown swan. The notion of such implicit coercion would revolt a contemporary player.

As the moneyed middle-class and the financial autonomy of women spread over the next decades, swinging kept pace. If 'wife-swapping' was widely associated with the more luxurious suburbs, it was surely because in the suburbs were found the first double-income, entirely nuclear families. Contact magazines and informal networks sprouted up on both sides of the Atlantic.

9

AN ANOMALOUS ORGY

OCCASIONALLY, SWINGING RAN into independent but related cultures.

The hippy movement widely advocated 'free love', a notion which swingers largely reject. Whilst the more idealistic hippies cut their hair and enrolled in banks and oil companies or sank into traditional politics, many of those of more radical and practical bent who espoused feminism and libertarianism became not only, *inter alia*, the founding fathers and mothers of modern pornography but some of the most influential figures in the mainstream media, the arts and academe. Many of these became swingers.

So hippies did not swing, but many swingers were once hippies, read hippies' books or attended hippies' seminars.

And again, I was taken to my first *partouze* in Paris as a student in the late '70s. Was this an early continental form of swinging or a local anomaly? It was a very elegant orgy with just eighteen of us playing around a pool and in an eighteenth-century orangery-cum-poolhouse-cum-bar. The apparently haphazard method of gathering guests, all of whom proved slender, well-coiffed and elegantly dressed, argued a very well-ordered and exclusive group.

My hostess, Sylvie, drove my girlfriend and me some distance out of town towards Longchamps in a yellow Di Thomaso Panterra. Her husband Thibault travelled ahead in a black Jensen. He drove slowly up and down an avenue, exchanging signals consisting of flashing headlights with passing cars. Some of these drew in beside us.

After half an hour or so of such signalling, and without exchanging a word with those parked alongside, we drove in cortege to a hunting lodge where a sleek middle-aged man and his very gorgeous, honey-coloured wife were waiting for us – he in a gold-buttoned blazer and pale grey flannels, she in a gold bikini and red flared culottes.

Thibault, my host, claimed that such *partouzes* belonged to a French tradition centuries old and that his grandfather had attended similar orgies in the Bois. I have no idea whether this be true, but there were marked differences between that party and a modern lifestyle event.

First, this was *une soirée particulière*. For all the apparent randomness of the meetings on the road, the drive was now filled with cars as elegant and expensive as ours, yet Thibault and Sylvie seemed to know no one save our hosts.

They knew *of* several. There was a chic and imperious woman in her forties – apparently a well-known publisher or editor in fashion magazines – who arrived with a very much younger lover. I played too with a very pretty, freckle-faced singer, again apparently well-known to the French public. She was in her late twenties or early thirties, but her partner or husband had pewter hair and black designer stubble. There was a photographer in there too, with his mixed-race American model girlfriend ...

This was a jet-set social *milieu* founded on class and style, not merely on sexual preferences. In retrospect, those preferences were subtly different from those generally observed in swinging today.

Most of the activity was heterosexual. Each of the women there was rather lazily fucked in turn by three or four men – without condoms, of course – during the course of the evening, whilst other men and sometimes women caressed them and conversed urbanely, sometimes with others who stood around fully clothed. I felt that we were putting on a show.

The publisher ordered her own minor gang-bang towards the end of the proceedings and had three men shower her with ejaculate. Otherwise, there was no group-sex and everything was very slow, luxuriant and Harold Robbins – hardcore orgiastic fucking in softcore soft-focus.

With the exception of the American girl and Sylvie (who, although a Parisian, had long been a transatlantic air stewardess), who made love beautifully at some length in, and by the side of, the pool, the women were languorously demanding rather than predatory. They were on show.

My shortcomings – and they were many and very short in my youth and excitement – would have made me very uncomfortable in modern swinging. Here, I was cooed over and appreciated for my enthusiasm, affection and youthful ability to play repeated encores. I was a useful, novel and ardent addition to the mix.

These may, of course, have been differences ordained only by nation and era. France, after all, was a Catholic country, and swinging at the time may have been more exclusively the province of the aristocracy and the intelligentsia than in Britain and the US. Certainly on recent visits to Paris, we have encountered a lifestyle little different from that in London or Amsterdam.

Has an historic European aristocratic pastime, then, been subsumed into the swinging movement, or was what I witnessed merely a Gallic interpretation of an American import?

10

SWINGING IN THE '70S

ALTHOUGH THE SIXTIES – the era of mini-skirts, rich and rebellious youth culture and the pill – loudly proclaimed free love and promiscuity, it was a tentative time. The champions of sexual licence were the young. They would be the swingers of the eighties perhaps, but, save for a notorious few, the young in the sixties were not swinging. Brief periods of promiscuity or serial romantic monogamy before marriage constituted the nearest approach to a reconciliation of daring self-indulgence, self-interest and self-respect.

Swinging was spreading fast, but still largely within a specific middle-class, middle-aged *milieu* – the *milieu*, so often parodied, of now highly educated, often bored women (more and more of them joining the workforce) and their professional or businessmen husbands.

Contact magazines proliferated. Clubs grew up. Most of these were secretive networks which held parties in members' private homes converted for the night, but there were openly proclaimed swingers' clubs in New York, Amsterdam, London, Paris and throughout California in the early seventies.

These were in fact cocktail lounges or nightclubs at which swingers could meet and engage in more or less explicit sexual acts on the dance floor, on the banquettes or in the alcoves, but it was only in California that there were openly 'on-premise' sex clubs with large spaces devoted to orgiastic activities.

It was to be New York's Plato's Retreat, however, which was to become the most famous of these. Plato's opened in the basement of the Ansonia Hotel in 1977. It attracted a huge amount of publicity, bringing international popular attention to swinging culture – affording it a certain louche glamour similar to that of nearby Studio 54 which opened in the same year – and spawning many more modest (in scale) imitations.

By now swinging had crept out of the closet, with academic acknowledgement and sometimes support, successful national conventions and a thriving, if persecuted, trade association in the form of the North American Swing Club Association (NASCA), founded in 1980 in response to the 1970s' boom.

11

THE '80S AND BEYOND

BUT 1981 SAW THE FIRST stirrings of panic about AIDS. By 1984, with the active agent of the disease and the means of its transmission identified, it seemed that a new hysterical Puritanism was about to smother the newborn swinging lifestyle along with open male homosexual activity.

All the gay bath-houses were closed down by health authority ordinance in '84. As it was recognised that heterosexuals too could transmit and contract the virus, Plato's followed in '85.

I have already mentioned one of the paradoxical effects of the AIDS epidemic. Safe sex meant more, and psychologically less committal, sex. The rabble-rousers howled for vengeance, but the pitchfork-wielding mob discovered the newly built citadel of sexual liberalism to have its gates wide open, and the ogre to be not only normal and human but considerably more dignified and responsible than many of its persecutors.

'Gay' men and women – at a terrible price – won sympathy, admiration and emancipation. They won for themselves, and incidentally for others, an implicit recognition that sexual gratification – even without procreation or state or divine sanction – was an imperative rather than an indulgence, and that diverse sexualities did not disqualify people from the human race or from the freedoms assured by law in a civilised society.

Swingers owe a huge debt to the gay and lesbian communities of that age. They have yet to be afforded the same respect and acceptance as 'gays' on the faintly dubious grounds that the one lifestyle is elective whilst the other is predetermined (neither of which premisses is demonstrable and both of which are irrelevant to the possession of freedoms in a free society), but the resultant openness to diversity has certainly contributed to the burgeoning of swinging throughout the Western world.

Sex remains a subject that occasions almost reflex responses of embarrassment, envy, disapproval or disgust as though it were anyone's business but the participants'. This is mildly bewildering. Consensual sexual activity between adults affects – and so concerns – no-one but themselves, and so is no more a subject deserving of moral judgement by others than is, say, choice of dress or décor.

I suppose that, since state and Church have thus impertinently interfered in personal choice over centuries, many private citizens feel that they too are thereby entitled to chip in their penny's worth.

Swinging will surely grow and become more openly acknowledged as a mainstream diversion and culture. It is, after all, a civilised means of coping with the decline of the nuclear family without sacrificing its best and most rewarding elements – enduring companionship, social stability and security for children and other dependents.

History, however, shows that freedom and repression, humanism and religious fundamentalism, libertarianism and dogmatism tend to follow cycles – the one giving rise to the other. Prophesy is therefore unwise.

It may be that we are simply enjoying one of those moments at which the liberties and privileges previously enjoyed by the few are granted to – or have been won by – a majority who must now be appeased. When bread and circuses become staples, our civilisation will become top-heavy and founder, to be overcome by a new breed of barbarians, hungrier, less just, but fitter to survive. People will then look back and brand our age decadent and corrupt and will regard swinging and the acceptance of homosexual activity as proof of our amorality and at once a cause and a symptom of our decline.

Until the unhealthily healthy, the heartlessly hearty and the liberal interventionist reclaim the high ground, however, I see little alternative to the spread of swinging. Promiscuity and infidelity are ugly and disorderly. Unevolved marriage, as currently constituted, is often repressive, unfulfilling and unsuccessful.

My friend Fiona – the doctor's wife, who maintained that swinging devalued sex – acknowledged the truth of this, but complained, 'Yes, but it shouldn't be like that. It was better when there was romance and fidelity in marriage.'

I told her: 'And dodos may have tasted better than turkeys, but, even if it were true, it isn't interesting because it leads us nowhere. And anyhow, *was* it better for women when they were all but owned, and kept indoors and obliged to have children until they died? And the plain ones must remain virgins and the unruly ones become whores? And men must deceive and transmit fatal diseases to their wives? Because these were the corollaries of the courtship market in which sex was dressed up as respectable romance ...'

This was a debate which could continue indefinitely. The society which I was denigrating and Fiona coveting had sorted things out according to its resources and its requirements, just as we were attempting to reconcile our natures with the conventions and provisions of our own time.

PART V

1

CYBERQUESTING

AFTER THE FIRST FEW PARTIES, and the discovery that we had enjoyed them enormously, Lisa and I started to look around for meets.

If the Internet has given dating a shot in the arm, it has galvanised swinging like a bolt of lightning.

Back in the mid-1980s, my then girlfriend and I bought a few contact magazines called, as far as I can remember, *UK Rendezvous*, *Silk Swingers* and the like.

These small-format publications with a slippery gloss finish on their thin pages featured standard, breathy pornographic stories, purporting to be real-life swingers' accounts of their experiences. The vocabulary, the imagery and the nature of the fantasies, however, suggested a solitary male at work.

When supposedly written by women, they tended to involve plumbers and gardeners who 'reamed' them a lot.

I have never encountered this verb in any other context. It means, alarmingly, 'to enlarge a hole by means of a reamer – a steel tool with longitudinal teeth' or, in the United States, only slightly more appositely, 'to extract juice from a citrus fruit'.

Anyhow, plumbers and gardeners, and – on one notably incredible occasion – a hairdresser and an interior designer, frequently reamed grateful women 'like stallions' and worked them like bandsaws, either behind their husbands' backs or with their husbands' collusion, until, invariably, the women had the most explosive orgasms that they had ever experienced.

Shortly afterwards, the men in question 'jetted' them or 'splattered' them with 'spunk' or 'come' (latterly 'cum'), which was invariably 'hot' and 'creamy' and for which the women showed voracious appetite.

When it was a man narrating the tale, he told of women who hunted in pairs and lusted after one another without the least embarrassment or even amusement beyond the cool, designing and disdainful variety.

Such women lay in wait and pounced upon them. Their lusts were invariably described in terms of wildcats, who generally had intercourse with stallions, who in turn favoured 'reaming' them. Again, the conclusion entailed splattering to shame Tarantino.

Interspersed with these stories were pages of small ads with black and white pictures attached and box numbers to which responses could be addressed.

My girlfriend's interest had been assumed and fantastic. She fantasised about having another woman in our bed. She fingered the dark fur between the legs of the women in the photographs, then licked her fingertips.

I have since discovered that many, many couples on swinging sites are like us – flirting with the notion in order to stimulate sexual fantasy and desire and generally getting in the way of real swingers.

Some few of these actually venture further and realise those fantasies. I was one such.

A psycho-analyst once checked me out. She said, 'Your problem is, you're a liver-out of fantasies.' I replied, I then thought amusingly, that actually my problem was that I *had* a liver out of fantasies – and gruesome fantasies at that – but that my tendency to essay experiences which seemed to me appealing or amusing was entirely healthy and, aside from the expense involved, no problem at all.

In *Silk Swingers*, I happened upon a couple in Hungerford looking for a single male. I wrote to them and received an encouraging reply with a telephone number. She was a barmaid who might easily have been called Elaine. He was, I think, Geoff, an ex-convict 'in the building trade'.

When I arrived at their little red brick terraced house, with a fallen window-box for a garden, I carried a bottle of Veuve Clicquot. She said, 'Ooh,' and produced a bowl of crisps. She was a pretty, slim blonde of twenty-eight, he muscular, dark, Latin-looking and ten years her senior

We sat in their lounge and watched a porn video for an hour or so. At length, despairing, no doubt, of my doing anything constructive beyond talking about her bar-work and her little girl, she laid a hand high on my thigh. I reciprocated.

Geoff at once said, 'Right? Ready for it? Good.'

He shepherded us to the bedroom upstairs. She and I fell onto the bed, kissing and groping at one another's principal concavities and convexities. She was very warm and loving. He disappeared, humming, to lock up the house, I suppose, switch off lights and the like.

We were fucking when at length he returned. He wore a string vest. He said, 'Nice.'

I was still at an age where I came frequently. I did so that night – condoms were not even considered back then. Meanwhile, her husband (who at last shed his singlet but wore white socks and nothing else throughout, and every so often, willy jiggling, brought a tray of sweet, milky, dark tan tea with Rich Tea biscuits on the side, to sustain us in our strivings) managed to do so once.

He said, 'Well, Gor, fuck me!' as he looked down at his shrinking cock in his wife's mouth. She looked up adoringly, licked her lips and said, 'Hey, babe! You see? You see?'

They regarded this as a triumph for which they were touchingly grateful to me. This was, apparently, a rare occurrence. They obscurely blamed his time in prison.

In the morning, I had a congenial breakfast of Rice Krispies and toast with their four-year-old daughter. Elaine stood tiptoe to kiss me very properly on the cheek as I left. She thanked me. I felt that I had performed a therapeutic as much as a sybaritic function. I felt good about it.

This experience did nothing, however, to make me feel that I knew anything about swinging. It was a pleasant, interesting sexual encounter amongst hundreds of others, many of which had similarly been the results of unexpected meetings in unfamiliar environments.

In those days, swinging – save for a small demimonde in the cities – was still 'wife-swapping' and, as its name implies, secretive, largely male-organised and far more an isolated, underground perversion than a culture.

Women might seek and demand sexual pleasure back then, but had yet to take control of a playground in which they could obtain it.

The infamous and wholly offensive suburban ritual (possibly mythical but suggestive for all that) of placing car keys in a bowl, then drawing them out at random to see who was paired with whom, was characteristic.

The Internet has changed all that. As with Friends Reunited and other sites which supply a community which would once, with the extended family, have been accessible, the Internet has brought this subculture or 'lifestyle' within the reach of millions.

2

LOCAL-SWINGERS.CO.UK

TODAY, THERE ARE COUNTLESS WEBSITES providing – at least theoretically – discreet facilities for swingers to seek one another out and to arrange meetings.

Many of these – though at first sight, lush and full of colour pictures of drink-advertisement-type girls in scant clothing – are in fact mere fantasy sites, and many of the women working girls plying for trade, or Eastern European models who neither care nor probably know where their images end up.

Lisa and I scanned several of these sites and could have wasted several days and hundreds of pounds had a friend of hers not directed us to local-swingers.co.uk. We at once decided that this was what we were after.

It is a reassuringly businesslike and efficient site. Its predominant colours are canary yellow and grey. Once logged in, you can scan the entire nation of swingers, location by location.

In Aberdeen (central) – to start at the top of the alphabetical list

– there are 308 individuals or couples looking for sexual diversion – 127 couples, 10 single females and 171 single males.

In respectable little Alton in Hampshire, there are eleven couples, two females (taglines: 'Does My Software Make You Hard?' and 'Single – sort-of – Looking for Fun and Laughter') and seven males.

This is probably more typical than the Aberdeen ratio. The largest category of advertiser is the couple with bi or bi-curious female, looking for 'similar or bi female'. Then come the straight (or 'str8') single males, mostly mere drooling hyenas grown tired of table legs and now trying their luck.

Then there are straight couples looking merely to share partners, bi couples seeking multiple, Man of Karthoum combinations, and single females, who enjoy all the benefits and confusions of a huge sellers' market. Of these, some few – invariably married – are merely seeking other women. Out-and-out gay men and women do not seem to use this site. They have their own fora elsewhere.

Every one of these profiles boasts a tagline, which may be as simple as 'Couple' or 'Horny couple', but, with the single men, often exhibits really quite startling want of originality and charm.

They run the gamut of pop-song and rap themes. Certain of them attempt to make a virtue of desperation: 'I Need Your Juicy Pussy, and I Need It Now! Yum!', 'Big Daddy Wants Your Booty', 'So What Am I Doing Wrong?', 'There Must Be Someone Out There ...'. Many more focus upon their author's presumed experience and proficiency: 'Everhard & Ready at Your Service', '200 Satisfied Women Can't Be Wrong ...', and even the staggeringly ignorant 'Great Technique! Orgasm Guaranteed!'

Another demonstration of ignorance is the obsession with penis size. There seems to be a deal of confusion here as to what is or is not an acceptable size. '6 inches of quivering gristle' may appeal to someone, and there is no doubt a woman somewhere who yearns to supply a refuge for '11 inches looking for a snug home'.

Close-up pictures of these organs, jutting vainly into space with-out points of reference in order to appraise scale, generally evoke revulsion, sneers or, just occasionally, pathos rather than lust.

The profiles list 'equipment' and 'breasts' in terms of 'small', 'medium' or 'large'. There are those who, although plainly concerned with precision, list their equipment as 'medium' and elsewhere state that it is a mere '6 inches' or even '5.7 inches', whilst others consider 7 inches to be 'large'.

'Someone Make Me an Offer Before It's Too Late' pleads a 52-year-old, portly married man from Scunthorpe, calling himself 'Hern (sic) the Hunter' and looking for 'Bi Single Male, Straight Couple, Couple with Bi Male, Bi Couple' and (rather surprisingly) 'Straight, but not Bi, Female'.

'Experience: Never Tried Before,' says Hern, who can travel, will travel, but definitely cannot accommodate. Beneath this, there are four pictures, all plainly taken on self-timer, of Hern's tubby tum with its scribbles of black hair, and, beneath it, a funny little puce penis which possesses undoubted character. It looks like a lost, bullish, shaven little terrier nosing out of thick cover. Lisa said, 'Oh, yuk!' but, then, of another, apparently indistinguishable to me, 'Ah. It's sweet. I sort of feel I want to make it better ...'

The single male is, in general, up against it here. There are some who are educated and thoughtful and have evidently made the moral and practical decision to renounce dependence and possession and seek NSA (no strings attached) sexual play. Many, however, see swinging as an opportunity for fantasy with the vague prospect of get-ting their ends away at less financial cost than with a working girl, and with less effort than is demanded by conventional wooing.

The huge majority of couples' and females' profiles therefore declare 'no single males' and, incidentally, 'no watersports (any activ-ity involving urination) or pain'. If these are perverts, they are very conventional ones.

Another feature on Local Swingers convinced us that this represented, for all its occasional infelicities, the community to which we wanted to belong.

On the home page, there was an 'in memoriam' section devoted to a female member named Naomi who had been killed in a car crash on her way back from an orgy that Saturday.

A book of condolences had been set up, and fifty or more couples had already contributed to it, expressing sympathy for the husband, who had been in the accident and survived, and recalling happy memories of the dead woman in life.

So, flicking from Naomi's feedback on the couple's profile to her book of condolence, I read, from the same couple, 'Great couple. Crazy, sexy, non-stop laughter. Great in bed and out of it. Naomi left us both drained, but we can't wait till next time,' and 'We just can't believe it, and our deepest sympathies go to Jon and the family. She was just so full of life and love.' From another couple, 'Lovely, funny, life-asserting couple. Jon knows how to treat a woman and Naomi is the noisiest, loveliest cummer ever. We can both still taste her – and like it that way!' and 'God, how can this happen? N was just such a gorgeous, bubbly girl. All our love to you, Jon, and please call us and come and stay whenever you feel like a break and the company of friends ...'

This combination of sex and death, lust and friendship was charming and assertive of communal spirit, continuity and an endearing realism. No doubt happy memories would be shared, tears shed and sympathetic embraces exchanged at a swingers' club that Saturday night before the mourners retired to the playrooms to assert life and mutual sympathy – and to honour the dead woman – in the time-honoured manner.

Pictures on profiles tend to be of women. These are usually sprawled on beds or staircases (a shot from the rear, featuring a black corset and thong, is the favourite), eating pussy or being eaten, being 'spit-roasted' between two men or, in close-up, with cocks in their mouths or – the porn standard – gaping like hungry fledglings, their faces streaked or dripping with ejaculate.

Sometimes they are merely gynaecological close-ups, which tell the viewer nothing beyond the fact that the women have genitalia. This, you would have thought, might reasonably be assumed.

Lisa, however, here revealed a prejudice. 'I don't like girls who wear it all outside,' she declared.

Er, OK ...

Pictures of men are few and again, rather pointlessly, tend to concentrate on genitals. With the exception of one, in which the erect penis is shown next to a can of Heineken, these give no indication even of scale.

In this topsy-turvy world, most advertisers, whilst displaying each last intimate crevice below the neck, are reluctant to show their faces, and tend to have black labels stuck across their heads in their photographs. As Lisa complained, 'At the very least they could show us if they look after themselves or not. Show me arms or stomachs or chests, not fucking willies!' She at once insisted on changing our profile to include the line, 'We will not respond to pictures of genitalia.'

3

TICKS AND FEEDBACK

TIMEWASTERS AND FANTASISTS ARE to be found here as elsewhere. Many *soi-disant* couples are in fact single men who will make appointments but fail to keep them. There are genuine couples too, flirting with the idea. Maybe one day they will get beyond making a date before discovering, usually at the last minute, that they have been unavoidably detained elsewhere. In the meantime, for all that we understood them, they were a pain. We once drove all the way to Cornwall for a no-show.

Local Swingers, however, has twin accreditation systems. When the female of any couple has telephoned the site, the entry is afforded a green tick. When the couple has received 'feedback' – or reviews – from others whom they have met, they are awarded stars, like hotels. This feedback is listed at the foot of the profile.

One acquaintance, for example, has the following raves:

'From L**: Nice lady, lovely tits and great head. Had me grinning from ear to ear all the way home. Highly recommended!'

'From J*****: Wow, what a lady. She loves cock big time and gives one of the best blowjobs ever. If you get the chance, you must meet her. WOW!'

'From D*******l: Every now and then, a great-looking woman comes along and blows your mind. Well, this one does your mind first, then everything else. Fantastic!'

'From K**** and D****: Really lovely couple. You both made us feel so at ease. Great laugh, great sex. We're looking forward to next time. XXXX See you soon, please!'

And some famous women have inspired mere drooling odes and sonnets ...

Newcomers are strongly advised to ignore all profiles without ticks and feedback.

I confess that I am as proud of my feedback on here as of most other achievements. It is a testament to a large number of things which I value, amongst which courtesy and responsiveness rank high.

Connections between swingers need not be established over days of conversation. If we were afflicted by a sudden urgent desire for immediate fun and friendship or find ourselves at a loose end, there was a feature called 'Swingdate®', which enabled us to advertise for meetings that very night. We were to use this twice in the first two months. On the first occasion, we met a couple of drunken louts from Exeter. On the second, we met and played with two delightful couples who have since become good friends.

There is also a busy chatroom on the site. We looked in on it, but did not join in. Conversations here concern family life, clothes, work, shopping and, occasionally, sex and peripheral subjects such as shaving, fingernails and fat.

The moderators here are attentive and responsible. 'I was on there the other day and a guy I'd played with called me "slut",' said our friend Laura. 'The moderators were on his back in seconds and I had to explain to them that that just happened to be his pet name for me. And if people try to draw you into private rooms without your consent, the moderators are shit-hot.'

4

CASTING THE NET

SO LISA AND I FILLED OUT the registration form, listing our status (Boyfriend/Girlfriend) and specifying (by ticking boxes next to an extensive list) whom or what we were, or might be, seeking (Straight Couple, Couple with Bi Female, Straight Female, Bi Female, Groups and Party Invites). Under 'Experience' we ticked 'Tried Before – Want More!'

There is a whole host of practices under 'Enjoy' which we could have listed, most of them fairly self-evident. At length, exhibiting restraint, we ticked, 'Straight Sex, Threesomes, Group Sex, Orgies, Adult Parties, Swinging, Oral, Role Play, Exhibitionism, Outdoor Sex' and, at Lisa's insistence ('Well, you never know,' she said) 'Gang Bangs'.

Can travel? Yes. Can accommodate? Yes.

Our personal profiles beneath these descriptions read: Name – Mark, Sexuality – Straight, Age – 47, Height – 6', Build – Medium, Equipment – Large (I consulted Lisa on this), Smoker – Yes.

Name – Lisa, Sexuality – Bi, Age – 36, Height – 5' 4", Build – Small, Breasts – Medium, Smoker – No.

As to pictures, we took them there and then – three chiaroscuro numbers of Lisa sprawled on the bed and one of us fucking, in all of which faces were obscured, then, with a 'What the hell?' facial pictures of us both. Then came the all-important summary. At length we resolved on:

'We are well-travelled, well-read, well-mannered, deeply sceptical and infinitely curious. We love to laugh and to enjoy uninhibited fun with like-minded people who can be civilised and know when not to be. We will travel the length of the country and beyond for memorable, sensuous scenes with people who know how to play and have fun, so anyone with a party, big or small, or a weekend or holiday planned, single bi-females or couples with bi-female who just want a day's or night's play, please let us know.

'Lisa is very bi and very greedy, Mark straight, well-endowed, well-travelled, imaginative. We love to laugh and play and get nasty – and to make slow, gentle love – for hours on end. No anal or water sports, just laughing, kissing, eating, sucking, fucking, caressing, friendship, sensuality and fun. Oh, and please don't ask what we want to do with you. We won't have a clue till we see you, hold you, smell you, taste you, and fully-formed fantasies never work out as planned. Responsiveness is all.

'Lisa is delighted if Mark has fun with couples or single women in her absence, particularly if he can show me pics or, still better, bring me his playmates when I'm back. I will confirm this if required. We just want real people (too rare in this scene) who know how to have and share pleasure and adventure and whom we'll want to kiss as much in the morning ... Let's play ... Sorry. Absolutely no single males.'

And, with the tagline, 'Sensuous SW Couple Seek Playmates', we consigned our fantasy identities – together with a £50 fee – to the aether, and our fates to the mercies of Britain's swingers.

5

DREDGING

THE RESPONSE WAS INSTANT, though not, of course, what we wanted.

Single males, illiterate or unapologetically disregarding our specifications, wrote in at once.

Some appeared to have read the profile, but to believe that the final paragraph did not apply to them. They ranged again from the uncertainly cocky to the frankly pathetic. Terry from Manchester told us, 'hay u lk like my sort of peeps n lisas bods just made for cummin on yeah n im the man to do it im a sex manic n megacummer with 7ins jus for u gal.'

A host of others, ignoring the request for responsiveness, plainly reproduced the same cut-and-paste messages regardless of recipient. 'Hi. I wondered if you were interested in meeting a truly gentle but passionate guy. Athletic and ready to travel anywhere to satisfy. Call me on ...' or, 'Nice! Wd luv to fuck u.' These were deleted as soon as received.

Then there were the 'couples' who plainly were not. 'My wife is a filthy slut who wants 12 guys to cum on her' was a bit of a giveaway, as were the hazy pictures of female porn stars, generally blurred because snipped or snapped from magazines.

Sometimes the men gave notice of their intentions. 'My wife is v hot and loves girls when she's in the mood, but our marriage is a bit dodgy at the moment, so it all depends,' wrote 'Sea Dog', 52, of Plymouth.

All of these were plainly aspirants but knew nothing of the Lifestyle or its mores. Again technology helps to sift the chaff. MSN messenger is the second essential resource of swingers. When we find a fellow swinger who seems interesting and amusing, we make contact through Local Swingers, exchange pictures on the Internet, then chat on MSN, on which real-time conversations and, still better, webcam, allow a brief 'courtship' before meetings in person are arranged.

• • •

Laura first signed onto Local Swingers as a single girl. 'I had hundreds of replies. I did my best. I changed my profile, adding a note to the effect that, whilst it might take a while to get back to everyone, I would try to reply to all messages save for one-liners and messages in textspeak which would be deleted at once.

'I prepared a couple of stock replies to speed things up but, even with just a quick glance at each profile, it took a good five minutes to reply to each message. I was soon putting in an extra six hours at the end of a working day, just reading and answering messages.'

She found assistance from an improbable source. 'My 49 year-old mum came to visit and asked what I was doing on the computer in the evenings. Slightly nervously, I explained what I had been doing and tried to explain my reasons for choosing this rather than a more conventional route to romance. I showed her my profile and my mailbox ...

'And she just laughed.

'She looked at my avatar picture. "Darling!" she said. "You're going to attract paedophiles! You only look about thirteen there!"

'Mildly embarrassed, I went off to make her a cup of tea. When I came back, she was sitting at the desk, perving at profiles and alternately groaning, giggling and growling, "Now, he's not bad ..." or, "Ooh, you wouldn't want to go near her without a length of stout rope and a miner's lamp ..." There was a long pause, then, "And frankly, I think I'd want to send a canary in first ..."

'She responded to cavalier, impersonal messages with a brisk note: "You really should make a little more effort, you know," or, "No thanks."

'I just shrugged, shook my head, asked her to be sure not to miss anyone interesting, and left her to it.

'A year later, she had her own profile on Local Swingers and has a great time, though before either of us goes to a party, we always check that the other won't be there too.

'I know it probably seems pathetic, but the statistics on the home page of Local Swingers did wonders for my self-esteem. I knew that some of my correspondents hadn't bothered to read my profile and would probably have responded similarly to a single female halibut or a likely-looking watermelon. But despite that, I was really chuffed to see just how many people hit my page. My profile received over 1000 hits a week for the first month or so.

'The best advice I can give to anyone writing a profile for the first time is: For fuck's sake, don't write much about sex. It can just about be taken as read that, if you are posting a profile on a swinger site, you enjoy sex, just as it can reasonably be assumed that you possess genitals which, though very expressive and attractive to someone aroused, are not really interesting over breakfast. Be clever and funny and, above all, individual.

'The best advice that I can give to anyone responding to a profile is: Read it, and respond accordingly. Treat the person in question as an individual, not as a convenience. I reckon a real poet responding to Local Swingers adverts would get laid every night of the year.

'After the first few months, the number of messages began to decrease. Soon it was down to maybe fifty a week. Now I probably receive about twenty or so, which is manageable – even without Mum's assistance.'

6

SDC.COM

IT RAPIDLY BECAME CLEAR to Lisa and me that we must become hunters, not rely upon others to scent us out and give chase.

We found four couples within a range of 100 miles who seemed attractive and whose profiles spoke of humour and gusto. We wrote them brief notes, ensuring that we referred explicitly to their requirements – though these had more to do with social than sexual factors. Within a month, we had met them, played with them and learned of the other site used by serious swingers. We took one look and at once joined up.

Sdc.com is the world's biggest swingers' site. Formerly a disparate collection of clubs, including Swingers Europe, but now gathered together under the aegis of a hugely professional Florida parent company, SDC owns its own resort in Cancun, Mexico, has 250,000 couples as regular members, and holds 50 parties worldwide every month.

Its website is in six languages. It is bright, clean, clear, informative and, above all, user-friendly. On Local Swingers, you have to read through lengthy profiles before clicking to see pictures. In order to see facial pictures, you generally have to communicate with the people in question and exchange pictures on MSN. On SDC, a picture comes at the head of a profile, and members have private albums which they can open to chosen recipients on site.

Swinging is far more advanced and emancipated in America than here, so the huge majority of profiles on SDC show facial pictures of both parties. By means of competitions, the site also encourages high-resolution and elegant pictures. It is a pleasure to look through the pages of often really beautiful people around the world seeking amusement and sexual partners. SDC also has its own onsite messenger service, which again saves time and confusion, and has links with 'adult' holiday sites worldwide.

SDC has the additional advantage for those of us who travel that it truly is worldwide. Before trips to Cyprus, Italy, Germany and Australia, we flirted with couples at long distance, found out about forthcoming parties and were invited to meet them and, on two occasions, to stay with them.

And SDC couples tend to want to meet. They are busier people, perhaps, than the British on Local Swingers, less parochial and more accustomed to travel. Where a Local Swingers courtship may take months, SDC members tend quickly to establish a liking and to agree a meeting within days or even hours.

Whatever site is used, it is essential that the females of couples involved should talk on the telephone before any meeting. There are sad men out there who enjoy provoking responses with no apparent motive save envy and malice, and there are, of course, couples in which the woman is only a reluctant participant in her husband's fantasies.

Webcams are also necessary equipment – not, in our case or those of most active swingers, for ill-lit and dreary sexual performances requiring more hands than the standard issue. But it is galling, as once happened to us, to enjoy persuasive and flirtatious dialogue with a supposed couple on MSN, admiring glamorous, amusing and natural photographs of both members, only to discover that you have just one interlocutor, and he a pallid, unshaven male, presumably making use of images of an ex-wife, girlfriend or passing 'escort'.

Once it has been established that he or she is in fact dealing with a bona fide player or couple, the single swinger is still well advised, like all those involved in Internet dating, to arrange the meeting in a public place for security purposes. As a couple welcoming other couples met on SDC, we were not generally worried about security, but still chose to meet visitors at a pub or hotel simply to obviate awkwardness.

7

HANDLING MEETS

SUCH MEETINGS IN VANILLA LIFE are structured by convention. Guests are generally known to their hosts before arrival. They will enjoy drinks, conversation and games until a meal is announced and served. Having eaten, they will depart.

Or, again, they will be invited for the weekend only after it has been ascertained that they share a taste for tennis, shopping, horse-racing, stalking or whatever, or with a specific function in mind.

A swingers' meeting is founded upon the supposition that all involved love sex, has a hoped-for but far from assured purpose, but is wholly unstructured. Since no gong can sound to announce the transition to the next stage as if for dinner, shuffling, embarrassing pauses may result.

In the case of an evening meet, you have met, shared a drink and chatted about common friends or experiences. You have resolved that the visitors are attractive to you – or not.

In many ways, it is easier if there is no attraction and sex is not going to result from the meeting. Then the hosts or the visitors can announce amiably enough that, although this is all great fun and of course we hope to see you again soon, the chemistry just isn't quite there. Resentment may rarely result, but a public meeting-place contains the less discreet and supplies distractions. For this reason, many swinging couples will swear that they never play on a first meeting. This is often untrue, but it allows them to deliver a gentle rejection at long range after everyone has returned home.

If there is mutual attraction, it is altogether trickier. Again it is best left to the girls to get things going.

Say that you have met a couple in a hotel and shared a couple of drinks. Most swinging couples have already arranged a set of coded signals whereby each can indicate to the other that he or she is happy to take things further. It is less easy, however, to know what the other couple has decided, and no one wishes to be the first to express willingness to proceed.

If, therefore, the women can find an opportunity to compare notes, then start playing with one another or with the men on their return, or can simply declare, as Lisa would, 'Right. I'm fed up with this. Let's go home and fuck,' lengthy silences and misapprehensions can be avoided.

Very few couples want to share their beds overnight with visitors and to wake up beside them in the morning. Sleeping arrangements, therefore, or a time of departure, should be indicated from the outset. We kept a king-sized mattress which could be laid out on the living-room floor for play, so that we – and overnight guests – could resort to our respective beds when and if tired.

Casual meetings with locals were less consistently successful than those arranged at longer range. There were people who did not resemble their profiles or had omitted some detail, which we found salient but they had plainly considered unimportant, such as twenty years and six unnoticed stone in weight since their pictures were taken.

We suffered nothing so alarming as one Midlands couple of our acquaintance, who drove two hundred miles to meet a charming couple with whom they had corresponded at some length.

Unfortunately their correspondents had given no indication that he suffered from cerebral palsy and would greet them at the door clad only in dirty trainers and socks, nor that she was seven months pregnant.

There are always people too who write proposing that you play parts in fantasies clearly set in stone. A Basingstoke couple called Fred and Louise, for example, wrote more than a thousand words outlining their plan to have Fred and me drag Lisa to a tree, tie her up and have sex with her before Louise surprised us, whipped Lisa and joined in the fun.

This fantasy was so clearly formed in their heads (they had already chosen the tree, bought the whips, the costumes and the strap-on with which Louise would fuck Lisa) and took so little account of who we might be, of the mood, the weather, flies, thistles and other rather pertinent variables that it was clearly impossible to fulfil and, we discovered, rather insulting. So we left them to the pursuit of their impossible dream.

Because SDC couples travel further than the Local Swingers variety, we often invited them for weekends.

Only once did we make the mistake of doing so without ensuring that there was a party in the neighbourhood on the Saturday night.

On that occasion, Lisa discovered within ten minutes of their arrival that his table-manners and personal habits disgusted her, whilst I was repelled by the visiting woman's abrasive voice and bigotry.

It was easy enough to blame fatigue and a lingering cough for a failure to play that night, but the following afternoon and evening were thoroughly uncomfortable, particularly since the visitors were townies to whom the only non-sedentary amusements involved sex or shops.

A party on the Saturday, however, makes everything easy. If all concerned get on, you can play on the Friday, spend the Saturday companionably together, enjoying a playful anticipatory siesta in the afternoon, move onto the party as a foursome and return home, with or without new friends met there, to continue the fun. I have spent so many languorous, luxuriant late Sunday mornings with guests to the sound of the *Archers* omnibus that the theme tune now acts upon me as an instant, if incongruous, aphrodisiac.

If, however, the participants are not mutually attracted or simply not in the mood, there is still the party to look forward to. There are preparations to be made. The visitors are bound to meet someone with whom they can play, and you can stay long enough to plead fatigue on your return.

In fact, this has happened rarely. Such weekends have generally been spent – just as if we were regular humans – in showing guests the sights, going to the races, walking the dogs, sea-fishing and other pleasant pastimes in amongst the sexual games.

Sometimes these leisure activities and sex coincide. Swingers, like all tourists, like to keep records, and there are many pictures and films of us playing on boats, on the moors, by riversides and at ruined castles, for example. We have made many friends by this means, and have often returned our guests' visits.

In this regard, swinging is one of the few remaining activities that creates a nationwide – even worldwide – network such as our parents and grandparents knew in their social lives. They stayed with friends or had guests for sporting events, shooting parties, weddings and the like throughout the year. In my youth, I too would stay in strangers' houses for nearby dances all over the country.

Swinging opens up the same sort of social life for its practitioners.

8

ODDITIES ...

WE MET SOME ODD COUPLES in there as well. There was the curious pair from Leicester who booked a hotel room near Wells in order to entertain us.

We met in the bar downstairs. Tania was a primary-school teacher, Clive an IT consultant. They were unfashionably dressed but physically attractive – both kick-boxers and practitioners of t'ai chi – both caring, interested in the world about them and the plights of its inhabitants, both gentle. If they had a certain sense of humour deficit and looked at us with tender concern when we made jokes, what of it?

He was in his late thirties, she in her late twenties. They were fresh-faced, tooth-achingly nice and touchingly sincere about everything. She barely spoke. She was, he told us and she confirmed with a nod, 'very shy'.

They had started swinging for a strange reason. She had been a virgin when they met. He had wanted to marry her, but was convinced that she would soon begin to ask herself what she had been missing, so suggested that he accompany her on her journey of exploration.

She had no doubt responded with a hesitant, 'If you really think so, darling'. She had certainly read up on all the sociology, demographics and psychology of swinging, and could substantiate his points with facts and figures at every opportunity.

Her shyness did not extend beyond the bedroom door.

It was like Little Voice on stage. Tania was ravenous, uncontrollable. She guzzled and slavered all three of us. She whimpered and whined and yapped and keened like a saw shearing metal. She dribbled and drooled. She grunted and gasped and grabbed everything which came within reach and waffled on it, sat on it, or nuzzled into it. She was tender but insistent between Lisa's thighs and mine, and creaked with our every least movement.

Clive was something of an irrelevancy. He was poorly endowed and excessively excited. Within half an hour he was a spent force. She, Lisa and I, however, spent the next three or four hours in play, though we frequently had to pin Tania down forcefully.

Afterwards, she relaxed between us and began to talk more freely.

'Oh, I do like her,' she whispered to Lisa over her shoulder at one point. 'So hot. Tastes so good ...'

'Her?' I said. 'Lisa?'

Tania kissed me and looked coy. Her mouth wriggled. 'Well, yes ...' She turned her head again to Lisa. 'You know ...'

'No ...'

She reached behind her to finger between Lisa's legs. 'Her,' she said. 'Your ... Her ... you know ...' Her lips worked. Her fist arose to cover her writhing mouth. '... front bottom ...'

Here was a woman who had been fucked by two men and a woman and had swallowed two men's ejaculate, who had shoved toys up Lisa and herself before sucking them clean, and had spent hours lapping at Lisa's pussy, yet – try as we might – we could not get her to speak the words 'pussy', 'cock', 'come', 'clit' or 'arse'. She just blushed deep red and squealed, covered her ears and begged us to stop.

The primary-school teacher virgin in her insisted that her husband had a 'thingy' and Lisa and she 'front bottoms' or 'pennies', that she had been spattered with 'men's stuff' and that, in orgasm, she had been 'bursting'.

Then there were the bikers from near Hereford who turned up in leathers on two huge *Easy Rider*-type Harleys. Weekend hippies-cum-Angels, Katherine was a midwife and a moderate potter and she and Niall owned a smallholding, a fishery and a smokehouse. They were sweet and sharp and funny but they did not care for beds much. They did, however, like cameras and costumes quite a lot.

One day they drove us out onto Exmoor where we played in a ruined bothy, in a very wet bog and on a drystone wall – each of us in turn entrusted with the video camera as Katherine thought best. That night we went to Secrets. On our return to the cottage with another couple in the early hours, Katherine took a fancy to the light in a straw-laid loose-box. The following day, skin prickling from the straw, it was the boat and the naturist beach at Downderry.

When they invited us to stay with them, it was to a jam-packed long weekend of locations – a tower, a disused church, a cricket pavilion, complete with singularly cold roller. Katherine was called away from the pavilion for a birth. She pulled a coat on over a satin corset, entrusted her huge, flower-decked picture hat to Lisa, told us, 'You guys keep going,' and headed off to attend to another vagina performing other functions.

There was the couple with a luxury flat off Piccadilly – he an expat Israeli banker, she a French former model, now a boutique owner – who had a very tall, charming, elegant, funny but totally impassive posh English secretary who filled our glasses, suggested tea and biscuits and even came in with telephone messages and questions about meetings as the four of us played naked on the bed. She was plainly very used to all this. She delivered the line: 'It may sound like a silly question, but what – well, what else – would anyone like to eat tonight?'

There was a couple of police officers, a couple of farmers, a couple of singers who worked the cruise liners, a racehorse trainer and his wife, an army major and his wife, an orchestral fiddler and her trumpeter husband ... There are all sorts in the Lifestyle. We got on with them all. Good, amusing sex really makes it very easy to get on with people – certainly a lot more effectively than getting on with people makes for good sex ...

And then there was the Night of the Exploding Penis.

By now, Lisa had at last set off on her long journey eastward and Sally had joined me as a partner. We were visiting a couple in Mortimer, near Reading. Another couple had been invited.

We had all enjoyed a good dinner and repaired first to the rug in front of the fire, then to the couple's marital bed. Our host Paul – like his wife, some sort of high-powered City banker – was fucking Sally when first he noticed heat and copious liquid where it should not be. He looked down at his condom, aghast, and said, 'Is that you? What's happening? Oh, my God ...'

'It's not me,' Sally assured him. 'It's you ...'

'Oh, my God ...' he murmured again. He pulled off the condom with a snap. Sally and Suzanne, our hostess, squealed and drew back their legs. Paul murmured 'Oh, my *God!*' again, then yelped. 'Oh, fuck! What the fuck is ...?'

His still erect cock was pumping gouts of blood onto the bed.

The other couple who had been playing with us after dinner, but had since retired to their own room, now rushed in. Confusion was general as everyone reached for knickers and socks. Paul pulled six snuff handkerchieves from a drawer and wrapped his genitals in them before tentatively pulling on his trousers. We piled into the car and set off for Reading General Hospital.

Paul was convinced that he was about to die of blood loss. Had his injured member remained engorged as at first, he might even have been right. He repeatedly made calculations. 'It's eight pints in the body, right? And I must have – that must have been two just on the bed ... And say I've lost another two on the way ... I may have two pints left by the time we arrive ...'

We had grabbed the nearest clothes to hand – those which we had worn earlier in the evening – so Sally tottered into the huge hospital atrium in just a tight, black, sparkly see-through minidress and black holdups without bra or panties, Suzanne in a tiny blue latex skirt and matching bra. Linda, the other female guest, had simply pulled on a black t-shirt with 'I ♥ cock' emblazoned across her breasts and a little white satin dressing gown. She was barefoot. The other girls wore high stilettos. Paul, meanwhile, had a groin bulging with sodden, rolled-up handkerchieves.

We made our way between ranks of waiting patients to the main desk, where a gaunt blonde auxiliary refused to deign to look up at us. Eventually Paul announced, 'I am bleeding to death. Could someone do something about it, please?'

The woman reluctantly acknowledged our presence. 'We'll just have to fill in a few details ...' she said. She reached for a form.

Linda and Sally took Paul off to sit him down, examine his cock and reassure him. Dom, Linda's husband, went off to find coffee. I remained with Suzanne as she answered the questions put to her. Name, address, age ...

'And what is the nature of the injury complained of?' asked the impassive woman at the desk.

'He's bleeding heavily from his cock,' said Suzanne.

'Penis, shall we say?'

'Cock, dick, penis ... Do you know? I really really, *really* don't care!' Suzanne said loudly. 'You see, he is losing a great deal of blood.'

'And how was the injury sustained?'

'He was fucking.'

'I think "making love" is probably better,' said the woman.

'No, it's not,' said Suzanne, obviously deciding that this was her semantic *no paseran* moment. 'If we're being precise, he was fucking. He was absolutely not making love.'

There was a murmur from the people in the chairs behind us. The gaunt woman looked a little less sure of herself. 'Intercourse, then ...' she said hurriedly.

'Intercourse, if woefully imprecise, is fine,' said Suzanne. 'Now, please can we see a doctor ...?'

But, much to Paul's distress and astonishment, we were compelled to sit down and wait our turn.

After forty minutes, during which Paul very seriously estimated that he must now have lost all but a quarter pint of his blood – which, he claimed, was now located at his left temple and its adjacent ear, but which he could feel dripping continuously down to his groin – Suzanne and he were ushered into a screened off area. Before the screen was pulled across, we saw a bespectacled male nurse showing him to a black vinyl-covered bed-cum-trolley.

The ensuing dialogue, of which we heard snatches, conjured interesting pictures. Paul and Suzanne filled in the details later.

'Oh, yeah. Have to put a stitch in that,' said the nurse casually. 'See a fair bit of this, actually. Catholics mostly.'

'*What?*'

'Dunno why, but yeah. Happens to Catholics a lot.'

'Oh, my God,' Paul growled. 'Yep. Par for the course. My cock and life are now in the hands of a congenital idiot. Figures. Anyhow, how long will this take to heal?'

'No naughties for a good ten days, I'm afraid. This your lady wife?'

'This is my wife, yes ...'

'Mmm. Well, love, off games for a while. Sorry. If ever this happens again, just grip the vein tightly for twenty minutes and it'll heal itself. Right ...'

'Hold on. Hold it right there. Are you trying to be funny? What the fuck are you doing with that thing, man?'

'Well, you'll need a little anaesthetic ...'

'You're joking! That's a horse syringe ... You're not coming near me with that ... No! Where are you going to stick it? Oh, for Christ's sake, you can't!'

'Ah, don't worry. You'll only feel a little prick ...' (sniggers)

'You ... No, Suze! Stop the bastard! Aaaaaah! FUCK!'

'There. Not so bad, was it? Now just a leetle bit of *petit point*. The stitch'll melt away. Here you go ... Tell you what ... I'll put a little bow in it, shall I?'

I wish that I could say that we were more solicitous than the nurse. In fact, we all played in front of Paul that night and the following morning whilst he groaned in frustration and on one occasion threw a full bottle of water at Sally, Suzanne and me, soaking us but failing to dampen our ardour.

And we knew, if his City colleague's never did, that Paul set off to the City on Monday morning to handle millions of pounds for pension funds with a dainty little bow at the tip of his penis, his blustering pride perhaps a little bruised – and his testicles very sore.

9

... AND OCCASIONAL PERILS

ONLY ONCE DID I HEAR of a swinger who felt less than safe on a meet. It was her own fault.

Victoria was just 29 when she received a fastidiously courteous message from a man who claimed to be 46. He lived close to her home in Basingstoke, and his pictures showed a smiling, avuncular sort of face which might well be of that age and a muscular body gone slightly soft, not so much from neglect as from a relaxation of a once more gruelling regime. He called himself 'Bingo' and claimed to have been in the police and now to run a small security firm.

'In his MSN chat, he seemed all sensible and homely and full of good grandpa sort of advice. His story was sad too.

'He'd been married, he said, to a woman who had become frustrated when he retired and settled near Andover, so she'd insisted on swinging. He hadn't really wanted to, but he'd joined in just to humour her, and they'd made some good friends in the swingset.

'Unfortunately, his wife had broken all the rules and had fallen for a younger guy and, one morning, she'd simply refused to leave with her husband. She'd just moved in with the young guy and his girl-friend.

'So poor old Bingo had been left alone and was still in love with his wife, even though she denied him access to his children and had taken him for half his house and his hard-earned pension into the bargain.

'Now he didn't want any more exclusive emotional relationships, but he loved women, so he was trying swinging on his own ...

'He proposed a meeting at a winebar that I knew close to home, so what was there to lose? I could always just turn up and say "Hi" and have a drink, then go ...

'The first shock was that he was at least 20 years older than he had claimed. The photographs he had posted were of him all right, but it was a him when I was in bobbysocks. He had flappy jowls now and scrotal sacs under his eyes.

'I should have walked out right then, but OK, I have a weakness for older men, and Bingo – real name, George – seemed sweet. He was dressed as he should be – not in an England football shirt and trackie bottoms or jeans and trainers, but you know, well-pressed blue and white shirt, fawn trousers, deck shoes ... His waistline had sagged a bit, but he appeared fit and he was polite and attentive and easily amused. I had no intention of playing with him, but, when he ordered a second glass of kir for me and of orange juice for himself, I was enjoying myself and it was OK.

'Then his mobile shrilled. He apologised and wandered over to the door onto the street as he spoke to whoever it was.

'When he came back, he said, "I am sorry. That was this couple down the way whom I've been trying to meet up with for ages. They asked us to pop over, but I told them you wouldn't be interested."

'I don't like people speaking for me, so like an idiot, I said, "Why? What's wrong with them?"

'"Nothing! They seem great!" He looked all glum. "No, it's just typical bad luck that they finally get in touch on the same day as you and I meet up."

"'Well, we could still meet them," I said sympathetically. "I mean, I have to get back in good time tonight, but you know, if you want to spend an hour or so over there ..."

'He was pathetically grateful and happy. You know – "Are you sure? I am so sorry about this. They sound really nice." He pulled out the phone again and tapped keys. "He's called Jim and she's Moira. Now, you really are sure?" he was still asking as he raised the phone to his ear.

'So we finished our drinks, walked out into the still busy, twilit street and climbed into Bingo's VW Golf. He kept telling me that it wasn't far and asked me loads of questions about me as we drove out of Basingstoke. I kept looking down side streets and assuming that we must soon turn off, but we were out in the country now. We passed straight through Lasham. I was getting anxious by now. Darkness was falling. The downs were spooky. I wasn't scared of the guy. I reckoned that I could deal with him, and anyhow I still thought he was genuinely good-natured, but this was no longer "down the way", and the prospect of being stranded somewhere out in the wilds with no means of returning home wasn't a nice one.

'I told him, "Look, Bingo, I told you I had to get home early. I thought this was just down the road. We've been going for half an hour. I'm sorry, but this isn't what I bargained for."

"'Oh, my God!" He was all astonished, guilt-stricken, "I'm so sorry, Vicky, love! They're just along the road from here. I didn't realise. Oh, Lord. Look, let's just call in and then we'll head back, OK? I'll still have you back by eleven, I guarantee. Please don't worry, honest ..."

'At last, in a village on the other side of Alton, he pulled up outside a grubby little semi-detached former farm labourer's cottage. It seemed sort of appropriate when our host came out to greet us. His hair was white and flossy. It splashed up and out like someone had dropped a large pink round stone in the middle, and the top of the stone was still visible. A froth of white hair had also been forced from his ears and nostrils.

'He wore a thick, checked shirt tucked especially deep and hard into his faded brown cords, and tartan carpet slippers, for fuck's sake! He carried a torch. He leaned down to kiss me before I was fully out of the car. His cheek was all papery. "Vic," he said in a wavering Scottish accent. "We've heard so much about you ..."

'What? In a three-minute conversation on a mobile phone? With a man who knew nothing about me but my name?

'"Come on in," bleated Jim. Then he nodded at Bingo over the roof of the car. "George," he said, "How're you doing?"

'I was confused and angry, but didn't know what to do about it. I was shown into a long thin hall with old red carpet turned up at the corners and piles of old tabloid newspapers tied with string, masking the skirting boards.

'I was being steered into a sweltering sitting-room. The wallpaper looked like cold porridge with dried strawberry bits and a gas fire popped, and there was a picture of a sunset lake which reminded me of medical pictures of wounds. There were piles of newspaper here too, and a large television which burbled pointlessly in the corner. The colour was set all wrong, so everyone on there seemed to have overused the sun-lamp.

'There was clattering from the back room. Slightly to my astonishment, the door, which was ajar, had a poster of two snogging naked girls on it.

'"Is that them?" called this female voice. There was a bit more clattering. "Hi, George! How are you?"

'"Fine, thanks, Mog!" called Bingo from behind me. "Come and say hello to Vic!"

'So it was obvious that this couple had known Bingo for some time. I was seething, but didn't know whether I could hold my new hosts to blame, so, for now, I kept my peace.

'A woman came into the room. She said, "Hello. Sausage." For a moment, I thought that she was addressing me as "sausage". Then she said, "I'm sure you must feel the need after that," and dumped a dish of steaming cocktail sausages on the coffee table.

'She slung the oven mitts over her shoulder and gushed, "And you must be Vicky. Oh, how lovely. Jim, you haven't even poured them a drink!" She gripped the oven mitts again, bent down and kissed me. "You're just yummy!" she said.

'Her body was well-preserved. I'll give her that. She wore an outfit made of black PVC straps which criss-crossed her like welts from an ambidextrous scourger until they vanished into slick black, wide-topped stiletto boots.

'On top all of this was a little white head. The cheeks were shrunken but heavily rouged. The eyelashes were fake and long . The eyebrows had been plucked out and replaced with these soaring arches of black paint.

'And on top of all that again was a sort of huge mounting breaker of pitch black hair, shoved forward by a girly red velvet Alice-band, before giving up and straggling down her neck to dribble and wriggle on her shoulders.

'Drinks, in the form of a box of supermarket white wine, were brought. Conversation was jolly. Big Brother came into it, I remember, and football, and Bingo's work and Moira's period pains. Bingo and Jim discussed these and Moira simpered at my side and several times laid a long, ruby-tipped hand on my thigh.

'Eventually, Moira left the room. I heard her thudding upstairs. Jim looked at his watch. "Well," he said. "If our Vic wants to get back tonight, we'd better get on with it, hadn't we?"

'I stared. I looked at Bingo, who was smiling his reassuring smile. I said, "But ..." I may have said it three or four times.

'At that moment, a thin ticking mattress – bent almost double – a sheet or two and, last of all and pressed to Moira's breast, a couple of pillows, came in through the door. Moira staggered in close behind.

'I said, "No. No. Look, I'm sorry. I thought George told you. I've got to be back by eleven. I made it quite clear. And we've only just met, and ... and ... well, no!"

'They looked at one another with several wild surmises. "Ah, but Vicky, babes," said Bingo. "We were all getting on so well, and I never took that seriously. I've certainly drunk far too much vino to head home now."

'Jim started nagging me too, but Moira had dropped her burden and just stood amidst its debris, looking more bereft and tragic than either of the males. "But Vicky, hun," she pouted. "Of course we'd never expect you to do anything you don't want, but you're so beautiful, and I've so looked forward to tonight. We never get to entertain, and I'm really hot to trot ..." She moved towards me as if to embrace me.

'I said – I yelped, I think – "No! I said I had to be back tonight and I do. I'm very grateful for your hospitality, but this doesn't work for me and I'm out of here, so either you call a taxi or I'll steal one of your cars, but I'm going home ..."

'In the end, a forty-pound taxi-ride got me out of there amidst much pouting and recrimination. Moira ended curled up in the corner hugging the bottle-brush and weeping. Bingo looked accusingly at me. Jim shrugged a lot, sighed and continued making up the mattress on the floor, between the television and the fire. He at least was not going to be dissuaded from enjoying the second highlight of the evening – after the cocktail sausages.

'I reported this incident to the moderator at Local Swingers, I admitted that I had been stupid and accepted a ticking off. Bingo's profile was removed the next day.'

Of course, it is not only amongst swingers that such attempts to exploit people occur. The running out of gas in a deserted place, the turn of the tide on a boating trip, the same 'too drunk to take the wheel' gag – all are weary cliches of crass vanilla 'courtship'. The fact that these people were looking for a foursome rather than one-on-one 'love-making' is irrelevant. These were normal, desperate, amoral people who did not give a damn about the willingness of a sexual partner.

The same rules apply here as for any blind date. Meet in a public place. Notify friends of your whereabouts and call when you believe yourself safe. Carry enough money to get home. Never get into a stranger's car.

10

SAFER THAN TRAWLING

IN GENERAL, SUCH ONLINE DATING is a satisfactory and safe way of meeting new friends and sexual partners. You quickly learn how to weed out the thoughtless, greedy and unattractive. Then, after an exchange of pictures and flirtatious conversation on messenger, you talk on the telephone – always ensuring, if you are communicating with a couple, that you have a good chat with the female to ensure that she is real and fully committed to the process – and, at the last, meet in a public place.

All in all, this is a considerably safer and more selective – even a more conventional – means of meeting than the nigh universally acceptable process of meeting someone in a bar, having a few drinks, selling a host of illusions, pretending to a confidence that we don't feel, then returning home for a shag.

Laura has many such acquaintances in Basingstoke. 'They routinely get dressed up, drink a skinful of alcohol, snog a few men and take one of them home. Next morning – usually after pretty shitty sex – they don't even know the name of the guy beside them.

'In the meantime, they will have slept a deep, drunken sleep, leaving a stranger with the freedom of their houses, computers, bodies – sometimes even their children. By morning, they could be pregnant, diseased or worse. But they've done things the respectable way, the accepted way, so at no point will they have to confront the fact that they went out dressed in tiny miniskirts and tons of slap because they actually wanted sex, so that's OK.

'Us swingers, if we fancy sex, we admit it to ourselves, log on, run through our contacts on a swingsite, pick a man, woman or couple we've already chatted to on Messenger and give them a call. We meet for a drink. If we all like and fancy one another, we go to bed – or the floor, or the haystack, whatever – and generally have pretty good, interesting, sensuous sex. Even if, by some strange chance, a guy's given a false name or false details, I always have recourse to the website where I met him, which will have checked his credit card details and confirmed his identity. It's a lot safer than trawling.'

Swingers too, as already noted, are committed to safe sex.

There are exceptions, as to every rule. A funny little north African man at Chameleons in Birmingham, for example (who seems to think that cunnilingus consists in planting his mouth over a woman's genitals and emulating a palsied limpet), persistently attempts to have sex with women there without a condom. Unless he is totally immune to derision and disgust, he will soon retire from the whole scene and take up another hobby. Beekeeping, for example.

There are also a few rash swinging groups which believe that, in that they play only with one another and occasional invited guests, they can safely do so 'bareback'.

Whilst swingers are rarely 'unfaithful' or play outside the immediate milieu, it would only take one errant member to precipitate disaster.

The normal swinger's response was quoted by Laura: 'Do you eat food off the toilet seat because it's pretty and looks clean? Yeah, well, the worst you can get there is gut rot. Unprotected sex with a pretty person can kill you. Er, derrr ...'

Maybe it is merely that swingers have enough sex, and sufficiently varied, to avoid the desperation of so many vanillas, many of whom have unprotected sex for the same reason as that with which they justify affairs with married people – 'It was just too much. I couldn't help myself ...'

This is not an excuse which swingers accept or acknowledge.

Oral sex is, of course, invariably performed without condoms. Penetrative sex, however, is always protected. When a man is moving from woman to woman, even when the two of them are muzzle to groin, he must change the condom each time. I have used twenty or more in an evening with just three girls. Women are also well advised to carry a couple in their bags for emergencies.

Sex toys are also cleaned between uses. Sarah from Pershore was so fastidious – or paranoiac – about hygiene that she insisted on putting a condom on both ends of a brand new double-ended dildo. This is ridiculous, but indicative of swingers' awareness of the need for hygiene.

And then, of course, a contact made through a swingers' site is as aware as any chef that he or she is subject to review. Those who lie or cheat in their profiles or exhibit discourtesy on a meet will find themselves slated in their feedback whilst those who prove amusing, considerate companions and good lovers will receive raves.

Safer and more efficient, then, than trawling around clubs, this swing-hunting offers a far wider choice than a haphazard gathering or a network of friends; entails none of the morning-after embarrassment and difficulty in restructuring hierarchies which characterise the office fling; ensures that he, she or they will place no individual demands on you and will leave when requested; and, generally, ensures that you will meet a fellow sensualist and moralist who wishes to leave marriages and established partnerships unbroken and the horses nodding peaceably in their stalls.

Yet these bonobosexuals, simply by dint of the admission that they seek sex, are morally dubious pariahs.

Go, as the Americans say, figure.

PART VI

1

WHO ARE SWINGERS?

IT IS VERY HARD TO FIND a single constant about so diverse a grouping.

Most swingers rediscover vanity and therefore make some effort to hone their bodies. Some are grossly fat.

Most are in what was once called 'middle-age'. Some are young, some very old. Many are religious sceptics (though many espouse Buddhism or some other less dogmatic spiritual calling, and very few in my experience spurn spirituality). Some are devout Christians.

Many swingers never attend parties but meet others only at one another's homes. Some – and this is a rash and dangerous practice, inviting jealousies and emotional attachments – swing only in exclusive groups of neighbours and friends. Others prefer to meet at 'munches', or swingers' socials, in pubs or other public venues where no playing is permitted, but where they identify one another by means of fishnet stockings or some other code signal and – if they like one another – arrange to meet elsewhere at a later date.

Most swingers like to play. Some, however, will remain at least partially clothed throughout orgies, or will play only with one another and merely enjoy the view and the company. The sense of freedom from suspicion and shame is, for these, sufficient reason for wishing to be part of the subculture, if not participants in its defining activities.

'Even as we walk in and say "Hi" and clock the little frocks, the underwear, the insane stilettos and strap-up boots, all those flickering glances as others appraise us in turn, I just feel this huge weight dropping from me,' says Laura.

'It's just the knowledge that, if I want to sing, dance, strip naked, fuck, go down on a stranger, masturbate or whatever – even cry with relief and joy – I *could* do so without fear of disapproval or misunderstanding. I'm not saying I would, but I just know that neither my body nor its feelings and functions are considered shocking, unusual or obscene any more. It's OK. I'm OK ...'

From the very outset, there is the easy, wide-ranging conversation of equals and initiates. Swingers may talk openly of things generally considered taboo, but there is much more that simply need not be said. Where the sexual agenda is not hidden, it ceases to be a threat.

This is one of the principal social problems of contemporary life. We can no longer play (in the broadest sense) with one another when every unguarded action or word may be interpreted as a sexual signal and sex is scary, one-sided and taboo. Every encounter, every conversation between adults is political, competitive and potentially threatening.

Swingers have no such problem. Sexual signals consist of direct questions – 'Will you?' or, in Europe, in tentative caresses (in the US, even touching is frowned upon, and propositions must always be verbal and explicit). These can be rejected with a word or a shake of the head, invariably without offence given or taken. There may, after all, be a thousand reasons for such rejection, none of them inherently offensive because they are rejections of a specific request at a specific time, not of a whole person.

So it may be 'Not just now, thanks. I don't feel like it,' or, 'You're very nice, but my partner does not fancy yours. Sorry!' or 'Your cock is too big for me,' or even, 'Sorry. We don't play with fat people' – inoffensive because it's a personal idiosyncratic preference and because plenty of other people do and will – or, most commonly of all, 'Look, we really like you, but I think you'll agree that the chemistry just isn't there …'

Swingers do not woo by laying out their entire personalities, status, property and history nor therefore regard a 'no' as a rejection of their entire identities. They are all friends or, at least, fellows, and the request to play is a kindly and approving gesture, an invitation to share pleasure. Its refusal is no more significant than a refusal to dance or to share a drink.

So, swingers repeatedly testify, they feel free to talk with their eyes and their bodies, to laugh and to touch without inhibition or fear of misunderstanding. 'It's a very wonderful freedom,' says Sue, 39, from Clapham. 'It's also great to know that when we play, it's just because of desire, not thanks to artifice, pretence, costume or coercion.'

That nineteenth-century abomination whereby sex and romantic love are inextricably linked, and whereby a man is subject and a woman object, is erased. Male swingers play *with* women and vice versa. The preposition 'to' has no place here.

2

'ALL THOSE YEARS, I'D BEEN CONNED ...'

SOMETIMES, AS AT ALL PARTIES, hardcore swinging parties never 'take off', and everyone stands in the kitchen or sits in the living-room, chatting about books, television, gossip, clothes or relation-ships just like partygoers the world over. A few couples may vanish into the playrooms without exciting remark and drift back in again, hair perhaps a little disordered, dress a little crumpled. Occasionally a woman may follow one of these couples, leaving her partner chat-ting, and reappear with them later.

The fact that these have been snogging, waffling at one another's groins, gasping, grunting and growling and mingling sweat and saliva as they play the primal game, is of precisely no significance.

On the other hand, for no more apparent reason than that for which customers at a restaurant will order steak one week and fish the next, the same party may catch fire. Then the kitchen is mysteri-ously empty and the playrooms packed.

Sex, however, is not the reason for which most swingers attend parties, as catching fish is not the purpose of civilised game-fishermen. It is the heightened awareness afforded by the possibility of sex, the freedom in conversation which that affords, the freedom to dress erotically – even, perhaps, absurdly – and to strut one's fanciful stuff, the company of other socially conventional libertarians and – in Britain at least – the rare ease between social backgrounds and age groups which draw swingers again and again to these events.

'It was like taking off your clothes and sinking into a bath after a day of grimy work and travel,' said Kirsty, 41 – a Bristol housewife and single parent whom I had taken to her first swingers' party. In that one night, she more than doubled her lifetime's total of lovers and, having told me beforehand that she 'couldn't see herself doing that,' had had two women come on her mouth.

'It's like, "Hey! I can do whatever I like. I can be me. I can show my naked body and my naked desires and everyone's going to approve and kiss me and share that freedom and love me for who I am, not who I pretend to be."'

Kirsty is one of many women who, in our interviews, has spontaneously used the word 'cheated' or 'conned' of her past life. 'They told me I'd be damned. They told me there were just two sorts of girl – the sort that deserved praise and the sort that enjoyed sex – and just two alternative courses in life. Every story made the point. "Your genitals are shameful and dirty. You can't be virtuous and raunchy. Find a man and you'll be happy ever after, but you can't find a man and have a happy family if you're a slut."

'All that shit was instilled from the nursery onwards, and it's like total garbage! I left that party smiling and was smiling for weeks afterwards, and occasionally burst into fits of happy giggles, because there was a place where I could openly flaunt all the stuff I'd had to hide for thirty years. I'd fulfilled my fantasies and I hadn't been struck by lightning.

'In fact, I felt better and happier and more together than I had in decades. Even the kids noticed it. It didn't turn me into a monster. It didn't stop me having normal relationships. It just made me feel happy and gave me lots of lovely stuff to look forward to and back on. All those years, I'd been conned ...'

3

CLASS AND AGE

THE SWINGING FRATERNITY IS, to some extent, limited both as to class and age. Swingers tend to be middle-class or *de facto* middle-class in that they are graduates, sole-traders, small business owners, artists or those accustomed – albeit low in their hierarchies – to exercising some executive autonomy.

Just off the top of my head, I could name police officers, teachers, doctors, barristers, managers, business consultants, actors, counsellors and healers of both sexes, editors, nurses, male politicians, bankers, stockbrokers, financial advisors, company directors and rank and file of both sexes in the armed forces, who swing.

I could also name artists and academics, journalists, television performers and technicians and a lot of owners of small businesses – boutiques, garages, import-export, publishing houses, market stalls. I know of no civil servants, though I am sure they exist. In general, however, swingers are educated free-thinkers accustomed to working on their own initiative within orderly structures, rather than apparatchiks slavishly following rules.

This is unsurprising. Swingers have contrived to reconcile conventional family values and social structures – and often religious beliefs – with the conviction that teachings on sexual pleasure are repressive, hypocritical nonsense with no foundations in history, psychology, anthropology or medicine.

Again the age range of swingers is limited, though less so than many would think. I know eighteen-year-old girls who are regulars at swing-parties, but they are few.

Curiously, although some male swingers seem to believe that these represent a lottery win, older females tend to disapprove.

'At that age, they should still be making all the normal silly mistakes and falling in love and believing in stuff,' said Sally, 41, watching Zoe – a 19-year-old, golden-skinned Zimbabwean – kneeling on a mattress between three men. 'If I talked to her and she convinced me that she was really happy here and that it felt right, I'd be happy to help her and maybe play with her. But yes, something in me tells me it's sad and all wrong.'

That 'something' is, I suspect, Sally's maternal impulses. These are reciprocated in filial form by some of the young girls. Katy, who took up swinging at 21, declares that she would never play with a woman older than her mother because 'that would just be weird'.

There are even fewer young boys in swinging.

This may be due to embarrassment or the hair-trigger ejaculations of male youth which don't fit in well with the abundance of stimuli involved in swinging. It may be that young men seldom have relationships or social status sufficiently assured for swinging, or that jealousy seems to be an overwhelming passion in young men. It may simply be that the relatively few young female swingers (the number is constantly growing) tend to be free spirits and sexually demanding and therefore to fly solo or to associate with older men.

In the big cities such as London, there are far more young swingers than in the provinces, which augurs well for swinging's future. Fever, perhaps the ultimate 'metropolitan swingers' club, has an upper age-limit of 35. Its parties, held at a variety of grand and luxurious locations in central London, are invariably packed with limber young couples, many of them working in City financial institutions.

Here, where many energetic and highly motivated young people are deferring child-bearing and rearing in the cause of their careers, swinging serves much the same function for the young – providing mutual companionship, adventure and play to couples without other shared purpose to bind them – as it serves in other contexts for older couples whose children no longer require full-time nurturing.

The overwhelming majority of swingers, however, are between the ages of 28 and 60. The average age is 40. It is rare that people (and especially women, who receive no validation of their individual sexualities from their parents or siblings, and only questionable validation from the media and a small selection of lovers) are confident enough in their own sexuality before the age of 28. There is too an inevitable dwindling of sexual urges beyond that of 60, though many continue playing well into their seventies.

Within that broad age-range, there are of course childless couples, those with young children who must worry about babysitters whenever they go out to play, and those with older children now able to look after themselves or already fled from the nest.

These last represent the biggest single age-category – couples who believe in marriage and loyalty and generally subscribe to middle-class values but, finding the excitement gone from their sex-lives and their greatest joint enterprise diminished or gone, elect to share new intimacy and adventure together. Menopause also often acts as a trigger to women to start swinging.

'I had twice been married and twice divorced,' recalls Molly, a 59-year-old author and healer from Brighton.

'My children were grown, and married and divorced themselves. I saw them making the same mistakes as me and realised that I had brought them up to make them. I didn't want to date, with all the hassles and supposed obligations involved. I liked living on my own. Besides, it was assumed that I would only date older, single men.

'On the other hand, I still loved sex and realised there was so much that I had never done. I like younger men and I very much wanted to experiment with women.

'When I first realised that the change had come, I thought "Fuck it," put my battery-operated fan next to my vibrator in my evening bag, and went to my first party. I had my first woman at 54 and loved it. I've shagged lovely guys and women of all ages. I love the whole thing. Now 90 per cent of my friends are swingers. I have a great social life. I get better fucked than ever before and my children think I'm disgusting and mad. It's great.'

4

'IT'S ME-TIME NOW ...'

IN MY EXPERIENCE, 41 is the magic age at which single, divorced or widowed women seek out a partner to accompany them, and married women plunge headlong into the swinging world.

Again, this is unsurprising. In 1800, when so many of our romantic and sexual conventions were being established in fiction and received morality, average life-expectancy in Britain – the world's richest nation, and one of its few nominally monogamous societies – was 36.

A young couple, then, barely had time to earn enough to win the means and the right to breed under a strictly Malthusian system and to rear a brace of young to scant self-sufficiency, before one or both of them could expect to die.

Those who did survive, of course, found themselves components of an extended family within a 'familistic society', with an enormous number of marital and blood kin and many roles as providers, counsellors, babysitters, teachers etc.

Today, average life expectancy is 76.

Forty years have been added to 'for as long as ye both shall live', yet the contract remains the same. For at least two-thirds of those years we can expect to be sexually active.

Meanwhile, the extended family has gone.

In our 'individualistic' society – founded upon that short-lived and failed social experiment, the 'nuclear' family – we are expected to find fulfilment, function, validation and excitement from just one other person, with whom we have no common purpose but the plumbing and the mortgage.

When first passion and then children have ceased to be their common causes, a married couple is often just two individuals sharing a bed and a house – she (to use surely broadly acceptable stereotypes) no doubt with her work, her charities or her gym-membership, he with his work and his occasional visits to the pub, the racecourse or the river bank. But they share little or nothing save the bills, television programmes and a bed. Every day of such separateness drags them further apart.

Once, if working-class, they would have had their own communities and other generations, older and younger, to tend, but the state has usurped all such functions.

Once, if upper-class, they would have had estates to run and tenants to care for, and a worldwide, sexually and socially active society in which they had defined places. Today, such clear cultural distinctions have been eroded, and with them the societies that they sustained.

The middle-classes have always been isolated. In their urban or suburban fastnesses – protected by privet or Leylandii rather than leaning over the fence to chat to neighbours, dedicated to amassing money and respectability but rarely owning land and so employing few people and working with few on an equal, sociable footing – their marriages, once the children were grown, were glued by vows and love or nothing. Infidelity was always widespread in such existences. Family break-up has become more and more so.

So the brave – some would say reckless – who are fit, prosperous and lusty and still believe that their marriage is worthwhile and that breaches of trust are not, broach the subject of swinging – that is, of enjoying sex with strangers, not separately, but as a team.

At or around the age at which, two centuries ago, they might reasonably have expected to die, today's women gaze out over a bleak and featureless future. Vonnegut says somewhere, 'I suppose that's really what so many American women are complaining about these days. They find their lives short on story and overburdened with epilogue.'

Well, a lot of those women resolve that they will start a new, exciting story instead of an epilogue, and this time, they will be the heroines on their own terms. To quote girl after girl of my acquaintance, 'It's me-time now.'

If they wish no ill to their partners and families and have no desire for emotional confusion, this may mean playtime.

5

SWINGING AND MARRIAGE

SWINGERS TEND TO BOAST that their marriages are safer and more successful than those of most vanillas. I have known exceptions, but believe this broadly to be true.

A recent study based on an Internet questionnaire addressed to visitors to lifestyle-related sites (Bergstrand & Williams, Today's Alternative Marriage Styles: The Case of Swingers, Electronic Journal of Human Sexuality, Vol. 3, 10 October 2000) found that 60 per cent of swingers said that swinging improved their relationship whilst just 1.7 per cent said it made their relationship less happy.

Half of those who rated their relationship very happy before becoming swingers maintained it had become even happier. Ninety per cent of those with less happy relationships maintained that swinging had improved them. Overall, swingers rate themselves happier (59 per cent against 32 per cent 'very happy') and their lives more exciting (76 per cent against 54 per cent 'exciting') than does the rest of the population.

Of course, figures attained by such means are dubious, but the disparities are huge, and swingers' marriages inevitably include a deal of variety, mutuality, commonalty and openness about fantasies denied to most others.

It is always correctly – if obviously – stressed, however, that swinging will not resolve extant problems, and that any couple tempted to take up this healthy and amusing hobby should have a close relationship and an affectionate – even if stagnant – sex-life at the outset.

The sights and sounds of a partner enjoying sex with another are unlikely to promote closeness and trust between couples who rarely see or hear such sights and sounds in their own beds.

Any peer-review or verification of swingers' claims is pretty much impossible. Empirical observation suggests, however, that those who have been successfully swinging together for a couple of years or more can probably count upon decades of mutuality and companionship.

The craving for adventure and the persuasion that the partnership is the principal obstacle to the fulfilment of unfulfilled fantasy, are banished. The intrigues, the guilt, the difficulties and the loneliness of secret, illicit affairs seem frankly unattractive in relation to the openness, the freedom and the uncomplicated nature of swinging sex.

Swinging extends far beyond the meet or the party. A swinging couple buys and tries on play clothes together (some of the best lingerie shops open after hours and encourage play in – and between – changing-rooms, which gives a whole new meaning to the term 'shop-soiled'), plots adventures together, seeks out partners together, makes mutual friends through swinging and has the nigh infinite pleasure of reminiscing about past encounters together, teasing and admiring, replaying fantasies shared and realised and conjuring more for next time.

Assume, then, that a loving couple finds itself bored and increasingly estranged when the children attain a certain age and autonomy. Neither wishes to see the other hurt nor to sacrifice a hard-won closeness, yet both – confronted with an unconscionably extended lifespan – seek sexual novelty, social adventure and autonomy.

Certain swinging zealots will claim that swinging in itself somehow and mysteriously supplies all the answers to such problems. It does not. If no trace of respect exists between the partners, if not a single ember of the fire which brought them together yet glows, swinging will merely blow away the ashes for once and for all.

Our yet loving and playful companions, however, can – if they find swinging congenial – count upon years of shared social and sexual adventures, intimacies and memories to bind them.

'According to King (1996) one of the things that normally occurs in a relationship leading to changes in how we interact with our partners is sexual habituation,' report Bergstrand and Williams in the study referred to above.

'At approximately three to seven years into a marriage, it begins to take increased levels of stimulation to produce the same level of sexual excitation previously obtained by a glance or a simple touch. A couple that is receptive to new and different sexual experiences will begin to explore different avenues of shared sexual fulfillment in order to continue to grow together. At this stressful point in marriages infidelity increases and the divorce rate peaks. Couples who find a way to reconnect physically and emotionally are more likely to make it through this period. Swinging may be one creative solution to the problem of habituation – it provides sexual variety, adventure, and the opportunity to live out one's fantasies as a couple without secrecy and deceit.'

It may be, then, that swinging works best as a marital aid in that it simply prolongs the years of excitement and mutuality. By the time that a couple – starting swinging in their late thirties or early forties

– has tired of the lifestyle and exhausted their fantasies or vigour, they will be well into their sixties at least, by which time separation for no better reason than sex should seem sillier than ever.

6

TAKING OVER THE DRIVING

'THERE IS ALWAYS A DRIVER in any relationship,' says Eddie, a 48-year-old swinger from Exeter. 'I thought that was me till we started playing.'

'No chance,' says his wife, Maggie. 'He'd be at home watching the football now if it wasn't for me ...'

This is a story that swingers have seen acted out again and again.

The man of a couple expresses an interest – often joking – in the scene. A colleague claims to swing and has given him a domain name. He has read somewhere of a local party. He will tentatively bring it up in conversation, suggest that it might be fun to take a look ...

And she, in almost all the couples with whom I have discussed this process, will play along with the fantasy until it becomes potentially real, then baulk.

She recognises a threat.

She does not know how she will cope with jealousy. She suspects that her husband is looking for other women as replacements for her, and therefore – by a deeply flawed calculation – that she is somehow deficient. She is terrified to have her body seen unclothed in public. She is simply at a point in the month or her life where eroticism has become alien. She is convinced that fantasy should remain just that.

There are those who will maintain that females swing only as a result of male coercion. This is unmitigated nonsense.

It is, however, almost invariably the case that women have more genetic and cultural conditioning inhibiting them than men, and therefore initially depend upon males to lead the dance, to answer their questions (even to supply their own already known answers), to reassure them and to pledge that the rules will be adhered to.

These rules, which most people come up with spontaneously, are in fact the absolute recognised rules of the swinging fraternity:

1. All sexual activity of whatever sort is clearly consensual, and no pressure will ever be placed upon anyone to play against his or her will. 'No' invariably means 'no', and no argument will be brooked.
2. All penetrative sex will be safe sex.
3. Whatever personal rules are agreed by a couple before swinging (no kissing, no penetration, no anal, no male ejaculation – 'save the last dance' – etc) will be adhered to throughout the swing-session in question. Variations may be discussed afterwards, but not in the heat of variable passion.
4. Play is only play, and bears no more relation to everyday existence and attachments than does fencing to real war (which does not mean that fencing may not be passionate and fierce). There will therefore be no numbers, addresses or messages exchanged or rendezvous made save openly by the couple. Swingers are the sworn enemies of dishonesty and marital infidelity, and will break off all relations with a playmate if there is the slightest hint of secrecy.
5. The welfare and happiness of the other member of the couple is

at all times the swinger's principal concern, and his or her wishes are paramount. These include 'I've had enough' or 'I'm not in the mood' at any time in the proceedings. Swinging is intended to strengthen and intensify a relationship, not to dissipate it.

Once the woman in this familiar story has overcome her initial qualms and fears and attended her first parties, it is she who assumes the lead and insists on attending parties whilst her husband or partner shrugs and mentions something about recent developments in *Big Brother*.

Women may take the ball tentatively, but again and again we see them run with it fiercely.

They love, so they say, the easy companionship, the glamour, the dressing-up and the showing off. They cherish the acceptance and approval of their sexuality. They adore the sustained eroticism ...

In many cases, too, they love the freedom to experiment with their bisexual desires.

This may in time become a less pressing motive. Today's young women openly and uninhibitedly experiment with 'lesbian' sex play where previous generations were reared to regard homosexuality as a permanent condition – almost as a disease. At present, however, there are many women in their late thirties or early forties who have repressed all bisexual impulses and now, when the opportunity is presented to them, plunge joyously into exploration of the sensuous possibilities afforded by their own gender.

Above all, most swingers are determinedly ethical. They strive to preserve marriages and partnerships, not to break them. They want security for their children. They behave and dress respectably in their daytime life so as 'not to frighten the horses' or cause distress.

They scorn those who have illicit, deceptive affairs, risking their principal partnerships and the happiness of those who have not deserved ill of them. They frankly despise those who, having taken such risks and been discovered, mewl of 'true love'.

'Lust,' says well-known Somerset swinger Donna, ruthlessly and very aristocratically, 'is to be expected and needs no forgiveness. You just aren't allowed the luxury of being in love. It's bad manners. Nothing excuses that.'

In acknowledging that they want more from life than one sexual partner and a progressively waning passion, they are tacitly acknowledging many other factors. They are thinking 'outside the box' to find an appropriate response to the decline of the extended family, the resultant endemic loneliness and searching for a place within a fragmented society, the prolongation of active life, the development of easy and reliable contraception, the emancipation of women and recognition of our sexuality ...

They are not, however, rejecting the social constructs which they deem worthwhile – discretion, a secure home for children, an enduring relationship founded upon mutual responsibility, knowledge and trust, a stable society in which the wishes of all are respected.

They are, in fact, behaving precisely as free-thinking aristocrats – and their modern successors, film-stars and rock-stars – have always behaved, only with rather more regard for courtesy and convention.

7

THE SINGLE FEMALE

THERE ARE SINGLE MEN and women who swing, but a lot of neither is particularly desirable.

Single women are welcome at all parties and are flooded with eager applicants as soon as their profiles are posted on sites. If action were all that they required, they could find it almost constantly – but then, so they could in any nightclub.

Thousands of otherwise timorous couples purport to be looking for single bisexual females to enhance their sex lives. 'But how do you know if it's really both of them?' asks Katy, who briefly became a single female swinger when her previous, occasionally swinging relationship broke up when she was only 23.

'She may tell you on the phone that she's as keen as he is, and sometimes I suppose that she will be, but then why isn't she committed to swinging rather than just to a tentative experiment with one woman? She's not lesbian, after all. Men tend to think that sex between women is somehow different, that it doesn't involve the same closeness or the same power struggles as heterosexual sex, but that's all crap.

'If you're bisexual and committed to enjoying sex for its own sake, why not meet up with both genders and enjoy them both? Why restrict yourself to women? Too often, what that really means is that the guy fancies having two women and would be wild with jealousy if his woman fucked another man, and she's just playing along with his fantasy because why not?

'But afterwards, as the outsider, you just feel like a gooseberry, and you know that they're desperate to get rid of you and to be by themselves so that he can reassure her. It's a big mistake.

'I had four meetings with couples when I was on my own. At each one, I felt that I was there to perform a function, not to be a companion and equal, sharing swinging fun. If you want someone to perform a sexual service or fulfil a fantasy for you, there are skilled professionals for just that, and they deserve to be paid for it.

'On the other hand, I also met several couples at parties who invited me back to their homes and we had a great time and became real friends, but they were real players, and invited their friends to meet me, and I'd go on shopping-trips with the girl, get to know the children and all that. All very conventional and relaxed, just like any other happy married couple with a single girl friend, even if we all piled into bed sometimes.

'In general, though, I hated being a single girl at parties. All the unattractive men instantly hit on you. Even at "couples and single girls" parties only, you'll always find one or two slimy little sods who will sidle up to you when their wives are out of the room. As everywhere else, the people you want to be with are the happy, confident couples who approach you together and take you under their wings.'

As for the single males whom she met through swinging, Katy's experience was much the same as that of all single girls on dating or swinging websites whom I have encountered. 'I received thousands upon thousands of replies. Most are just randy, lazy, fantasising gits looking for a free fuck. Many just send a "cut and paste" standard message. Again, if all they want is a pussy, why not go and buy one like anyone else?

'So to filter through all these people, triaging them into 70 per cent "Christ, no!", 25 per cent "possibly worth another look" and 5 per cent "potentially very nice", and to reply politely to all 30 per cent who are interesting or very nice – because all of them have, by definition, written proper personal messages, so they deserve a reply – takes forever.

'Then half of the interesting ones are absolutely guaranteed to be timewasters just flirting with fantasy, and many of them will turn out to be liars or married or in partnerships, and I don't fuck cheats. No-one in swinging does.

'All in all, I got eight shags and made two really good single male friends in my solo swinging days, and both of those were long-established swingers who, like me, had broken up with their regular partners and enjoyed the society regardless of the sex. One way or another, the investment in time and disappointed hopes is huge for a very small return.'

It is not hard for a single female to find a non-swinging male to accompany her to parties and meets. It is slightly harder, perhaps, to find one who understands and respects swinging's conventions.

Molly, at 57, invited a whole series of 'vanilla' men who appeared civilised to accompany her to parties. 'I said, "Come along and OK, you and I will play a bit, but I don't want you to think there's anything special between us other than our friendship. All I really want is an escort." Easy brief, you'd have thought. Every guy's dream.

'That was the problem. It seems that, if you give a guy his dream, he goes berserk. They wandered around – an accountant, a respected historian, a bookshop-owner, all in their fifties – like perverts, eyes popping out of their heads, groping everything in reach. The bookshop-owner, whom I'd picked because he had nice manners and seemed a man of the world, just took his clothes off and lay at the foot of the biggest bed, playing with himself and fondling everyone who played there, until he was kicked out.'

8

THE SINGLE MALE

AFTER JUST OVER A YEAR of regular swinging with me, Lisa bought herself a new wagon and set off eastward on her long-projected indefinite tour. For nearly four months afterwards, I was a single male on the scene.

Luckily by then I had extensive approving feedback on both contact sites, and friends from previous parties who visited and were willing to accompany me to parties. I also met several women from Local Swingers and SDC simply by dint of writing attentively and, I hoped, amusingly.

In general, however, the single male is up against it. Couples tend – as we had done – to write 'NO SINGLE MALES' at the foot of their profiles, and party hosts, quite correctly, charge single males – if they admit them at all – a huge amount of money after a selection process which would shame a St James's gentlemen's club.

I was by then sufficiently well-known and established to be invited to three otherwise strict, regular, couples-only parties as a useful, courteous, non-intrusive surplus male.

Although I got to play at these, I soon started to decline the invitations. Playing was still pleasurable, but the exclusively social parts of the evenings – the swimming alone in the floodlit pools, the flirtation and chat in the living-rooms, the sight of others excusing themselves to go off to play, the obligatory explanations as to why I was alone – all made the experience uncomfortable and frequently painfully frustrating, like Christmas for the lonely.

Playing loses a great deal of its appeal with transient partners. That intimacy, that sense of companionship and shared and mutual pleasure are at the heart of the subculture and are its *raisons d'être*.

So find a partner.

This is not as difficult as many would have us believe. Not only did countless women at drinks and dinner parties express tentative interest but, out of curiosity, I signed up on two more conventional dating sites where I stated my requirements as clearly as was permitted. After a brief introductory paragraph, I wrote:

'I speak a few languages, am loyal, well-spoken, well-mannered, very affectionate, adore flirtation, sharing and play, but am fed up with hurting people who expect instant and total mutual dependence and ownership and who fall in lerv with illusions. You and I could both go down to a winebar tonight and drag home something niceish to supply solace or to ease needs, but one of us always hopes for more than the other and then there is hurt and confusion, so I prefer to play with people who know that they are playing, who like to strut their stuff, enjoy sensuality and companionship and uninhibited fun, then return to their orderly, independent lives until next time.

'There is, however, a vacancy in my life for one very special person (preferably bi) who will be my lover and best friend, who will play and feast at my side, reminisce proudly as we cuddle and make love afterwards and plot the next shared adventure – here, in London, abroad, wherever ... with me. To such a one I can be loyal, supportive and even – given our own terms – faithful. And after that, who knows? I don't close the doors against love in any of its many forms, certainly not with a close and beloved friend, but I'd never look for it as a first target with a stranger ...'

During the four months that I was on these sites, hosts of women responded. Some had read only selectively. They wrote declaring that they were looking for a Mr Right who, it seemed, wore shining armour (so presumably attracting arrows and demonstrating that he had never been in a fight).

Many others, however, well able to read between the lines, expressed their approval and wanted to chat. Some, of course, were merely curious and wanted to know more about swinging. A few flirted with the notion of joining in to the extent of making tentative dates for meeting, but vanished into cyber-silence as the dates approached.

Three respectable 'vanilla' women met me, all but dragged me – unresisting – into bed, had vigorous and noisy nights of sex then informed me that they 'didn't do this sort of thing', that they 'didn't really know what had come over them (sic)' and asked me to leave.

In time, however, I met five women – four of them 39–41, one of them 26 – all of them fit and avowedly bi-curious, chatting regularly to me on Messenger and eager to try swinging. All owned 'Rampant Rabbit' vibrators and used them regularly. All admitted that they had often considered the Lifestyle but had been unsure about hygiene, safety and protocol.

They all attended their first parties with me, having met me and played with me for the first time that afternoon. They all enjoyed sex with a woman and 'spit-roasting' for the first time on that night. All have since become friends. One returned to her husband. The remaining four are still in the Lifestyle.

No doubt physical attractiveness, fitness, stamina, cock size and the like all play a part in a single male's initial welcome, but his acceptance in the Lifestyle depends upon all those usual attributes for which vanillas search no less than swingers – good manners, attentiveness, good humour and, above all, responsiveness – surely the key to success in the playroom no less than in the living-room.

If a single man is lucky enough to be invited to a party, he should be helpful, funny, gregarious but non-intrusive. Like any nicely brought-up young man at a traditional dance, he is well advised to be particularly attentive to the wallflowers – the nervous novices and the insecure. He may not get laid that night, but not only are the nervous likely to ask someone trusted to accompany them to the playrooms when at last they pluck up the courage, but they will soon gain in confidence.

Above all, he should assume nothing. He is at a party like any other, and must accept, as at any other, that tonight's outcome is at best uncertain. His aim should be to circulate, to listen, to learn and to make friends for the future.

Even when invited to join a couple on a bed and lying naked with them, he should play it very cool, caressing her, going down on her or whatever, but always remembering that he is an accessory to their pleasure. Always ask her before presuming to attempt to fuck her, or – if such be your pleasure – before caressing him. The answer may be 'no' right now. It may be a shrieked 'yes' ten minutes or a month hence.

There is a select group of such single males, many of whom I count as friends, whose names are well-known throughout the swinging community. Their feedback on the sites at all times runs into double figures from women and couples who have enjoyed them. They are welcome at many parties and can readily fill their diaries with meets with couples and single women.

What distinguishes these from their innumerable unsuccessful rivals?

The answers are predictable. They are well-groomed and well-mannered. They are confident enough to be at ease in any milieu, without being so cocky as to take over. They are sufficiently cultured and well read to relate to people of widely diverse backgrounds. They would be as popular anywhere.

Above all, they swing as a matter of principle and for pleasures cerebral no less than physical, not as a means to get laid. Such men as these can very easily get laid. They count a night spent flirting, dancing and meeting people well spent.

They recognise, as so frequently stated elsewhere here, that working girls exist to provide facile physical pleasures, and that male orgasm is incidental to swinging. Shared sensuality, friendship and fun are its purposes, and the successful single male swinger will get on with the male of any couple as well as with the female.

He knows how to play.

9

COUPLES STARTING OUT

THERE IS NOT MUCH TO starting out swinging for a couple. It is terrifying, of course, and marks an irrevocable transition in a couple's life together, but it is frighteningly easy.

I never went through the usual – usually disastrous – process whereby couples start swinging. This entails frustration, fantasy and a large amount of drink.

Suzy and Max are typical.

'I'd had a couple of one-night flings with colleagues at conferences and I didn't much like how it felt, always having to rebuild from that, always knowing it was going to happen again, all that ghastly false jollity and uncertainty and deceit,' says Suzy.

'Our marriage was fine, but we were both fit and frankly bored. Our children were independent every way except financially, and we were still in our late thirties. Aside from minor triumphs at work, the annual holiday, the odd half-marathon and so on, we had fuck-all to look forward to.

'We'd talked about swinging as a fantasy stimulant to our own sex.

Max is that kind of man anyway. He likes the idea of me with other men and women. He'd ask me to tell him what I'd have them do with me. He had this colleague called Simon who I quite liked, and Max fancied Simon's girlfriend, Valerie, who was in my running club. She was lovely – I mean, not much to look at at first, a bit gaunt in the face, but a great smile and these brilliant blue eyes under a Pandora bob, and these really full, gorgeous natural tits that just needed to be played with.

'Anyhow, it happened. Normal dinner party at their place, a lot of drink, silly jokes, Simon coming onto me, me taking Valerie into the kitchen and saying "How about it?", then us coming back into the sitting room and each of us going down on the other one's guy. She was my first ever girl. I'd been dreaming of it for ages. I loved it. It was fun, and afterwards, when we got home, Max was hotter and more passionate than he had been since we first met.

'Then came the hangover, the nervous sort of not admitting that you loved it because that might be treacherous, the wondering if he's preferred her to me, all that stuff, and we decided that it was a bad idea and that we wouldn't let it happen again. I don't know if we really meant it. We were both just scared.

'It had been great, seeing Max having fun and letting go with Valerie, kissing him and encouraging him, having him kiss me and beaming with excitement and pride as the other two fucked me – all of that had been great, and it had been really good going to work the next day in a smart suit and thinking, "If only you knew what I was up to last night", and smiling at the young people who thought they'd invented sex and at the guys who tried it on with me, because I didn't need any of that shit any more. It just looked so silly and messy.

'But I was unsure where it was leading. It was like a window had been flung open and it was exciting but very cold and scary out there.

'To make it worse, Valerie developed a bit of a crush on me and kept trying to get me on my own, and Simon kept nudging Max and suggesting that we all go off on holiday together, which was the last thing we wanted.

'It took us six months before we decided to give it another go. This time, we went to a club – Utopia in Birmingham – and I went a bit crazy. I went into this sort of blissful trance – pussy, cock, pussy, cock, just bring it on! Hundreds, thousands. I just wanted more. Gimme gimme.

'And Max was just so proud of me when we recovered consciousness the next day, and my jaw and my pussy were sore but we actually went straight off to Chameleons for a Sunday morning session, and that was it. Since then, it's been the best social life I've ever known. Hundreds of friends, loads of exciting treats to look forward to and loads of lovely stuff to look back on when we're together ...'

Again and again, you will hear stories of couples who started swinging in a vanilla milieu under the influence of drink or drugs, and discovered only confusion and pain often far worse than this.

Sabrina, a 34-year-old GP from Watchet in Somerset, is amongst many who admits, 'My first experience of swinging was the death-knell of my first marriage. We were frustrated and unhappy and drunk and we tried it, and it just underlined everything that was wrong. I looked at him playing and I felt sick. He probably felt the same about me. We never recovered. We never could have recovered, but that finished it.'

Sabrina is now with a new partner, and they are regulars on the official swing-scene.

It is in such ill-advised, impromptu imitations of swinging that marital infidelity (as distinct from shared swinging sex) and breakdown are most at risk. One member of the couple, with whom rare sexual pleasure was enjoyed, may start calling and begging for secret, one-to-one meetings with another. They may even convince themselves that they are 'in love'.

In a bid for the freedom afforded by swinging, couples find themselves entangled in swinging's very antithesis – the deception, confusion, gossip, injury, jealousy and alienation from their partners consequent upon the illicit affair.

Better by far to proceed directly and by mutual agreement to swinging proper.

• • •

It may be that a couple will in time discover that they favour private meets rather than parties, but a visit to a club – with no expectations – will enable them at once to meet other swingers and to explore their boundaries.

There is no compulsion whatever – nor any pressure, save self-imposed – for a couple to play at a swingers' club. Many treat it simply as a social occasion with a particularly interesting and stimulating cabaret supplied by fellow guests. Others will play exclusively with one another, so discovering whether they can readily undress in company or suffer from paralysing modesty.

The large swimming pool at Utopia, for example, is frequently lined with couples who, whilst enjoying the view and the frisson at exhibitionism, might just as well be at home fucking whilst enjoying a little pornographic stimulus for all the physical contact that they have with other guests.

'We went seven times and met lots of really nice people and really liked their company, but all we did was find a corner where we could play together,' recalls Maureen, 41, of her first adventures with husband Jake, 51. 'We saw people we fancied and saw lots of things we fancied, but we just weren't sure enough to touch anyone else. Partly nerves, I suppose. Partly just how would we deal with the jealousy, and what would it feel like?

'The eighth time, we asked a couple to join us, but told them we were just soft-swingers, so we got to play for the first time and did oral and all that, and it was no problem at all. We really enjoyed it and felt good about it afterwards. So we invited this same couple to meet us in a hotel for a replay.

'Again we just did soft, but I was gagging for this guy's cock, and Jake had fucked me while I was sucking this guy, which was something I'd always wanted to do, and he was harder than I could ever remember, so we agreed that next time, we would have a signal which meant "OK. From now on, no holds barred".

'By this time, I had no worries about jealousy. I'd watched Jake eating pussy – I'd done it with him. We'd both kissed other people and come with other people. It was just good to catch his eye and smile and feel his touch when he was all fired up like that. It was him who was still worried how he'd feel about me.

'So I whispered to the girl I was with at the next party and together we worked it so he was desperate to fuck her, so I gave him the go-ahead. She went down on me while he was fucking her, so when she said "God, she needs fucking!" well, he either had to stop what he was doing or let me fuck Dave. And all the time when I was being fucked, I made sure I was making a fuss of Jake – pulling him out of her and sucking him, encouraging him, slapping his arse, sucking his balls …

'Pretty soon, it just seemed incredible to us that we'd ever had qualms, and we almost never do parties now. We prefer the intimacy of meets at people's homes or hotels, but we needed to gain confidence and learn what it was all about, and that was the best way …'

10

NOT FOR THE IMPATIENT

SWINGING IS NOT ABOUT ceaseless gratification of desires. There are frustrations in there too.

On many, many occasions, my partner and I have met a couple who have seemed to me delightful and of which the female seems in every regard desirable, only for me to receive a nudge or a kick and a quick shake of the head indicating that my partner does not share my feelings.

Or, rather, in most instances she does share my feelings with regard to the girl, but does not like the man in question who, unfortunately, is part of the package.

Unfortunately, many of the loveliest girls in the Lifestyle – as well as elsewhere in society – are attached to large, outwardly ill-favoured men whose virtues are no doubt visible to them as to their brokers but are less apparent to the casual observer.

Just once or twice, my partner has desired a man whilst I found his girlfriend or wife perhaps less immediately attractive. Whether because the difference in attractiveness was not on these occasions so marked, whether because I was rather less discriminating than my partner or whether – as I like to think – I was a gentleman and so willing to make sacrifices in the cause of the greater good, I cannot say, but I found myself able to overlook the newcomer's perceived deficiencies. On each such occasion, my virtue was rewarded.

But since we play as couples, and consent is at all times essential to enjoyment, when there is dissent, we make our excuses and walk away. Swinging is not, then, for the impatient. We have all known nights of frustration in which everyone around us appears to be having fun and the place is full of stunning potential playmates, but, since we cannot agree with one another about both members of a couple, we must discreetly fret, curse and play, if at all, only à *deux*.

On one occasion at AbFab – a club near Heathrow – Katy and I were playing together on a large canopied bed and the party was warming up all around us, when Jackie and Steve, a couple with whom we had chatted on the net and the telephone, approached. They were late because of traffic. They introduced us to another young couple visiting from Cyprus.

It is a singular experience, reaching up whilst intertwined and stark naked, to shake hands with people fully clothed and to discuss traffic jams and driving conditions. We all laughed at the absurdity. We continued to fuck. The four others sat down on the bed to chat.

They started to caress us. At length, the Cypriot girl was on her back in my arms. Katy, she and I were kissing in a wet cat's cradle of hair and spittle. My hand rubbed and slapped a plush, hot pussy through damp cotton. Katy's breasts were being licked and sucked by Jackie whilst Steve mumbled and hummed in her groin.

Suddenly, Katy's hand squeezed mine sharply. I raised my head. She shook her head and mouthed, "No."

I could not believe it. I very much did not want to believe it. I looked at her quizzically and crossly. The Cypriot girl was struggling to undo her buttons beneath me. She looked and smelled gorgeous. I returned to kissing her, hoping that, when I looked back, as I knew I must, Katy would have changed her mind, or that I had been mistaken in my interpretation.

But no. Light had entered all that sweet, slippery darkness. She was standing now, saying, 'Sorry,' mumbling something about her stomach, and I had to make my excuses and – in acute pain – step over the straining bodies and follow her.

She could not explain it. She just cried in the car and in the hotel room afterwards, bewildered. No, it hadn't been the people. She had liked them. They had been really attractive. It was just – well, one of those mood things.

Much the same thing happened at Secrets a couple of months later. This time, she thought that she knew the reason. I had left her alone whilst I went to buy her a drink. She had been approached by a woman in her late fifties or early sixties. 'It was bad enough that she looked just like my Auntie Lesley,' explained a disconsolate Katy, 'but then she spotted my top and started to talk to me about crochet. That was me finished for the night.'

And I was duty bound to accept it. That too is part of the swingers' code.

11

PARTY HOSTS

MANY OF THOSE WHO ATTEND private swingers' parties wince at
the £25–£45 admission fee for every couple, look around them,
observe the more or less luxurious surroundings, and – maladroitly
putting the two distant cousins together – conclude that they are
father and son.

If they too open their houses to an easily accessible target market,
buy a few mattresses and a sound-system and push back the furniture,
they too will soon be popular, frequently laid and the proud owners
of hot-tubs and saunas.

They are gravely mistaken. Again and again we have seen such
parties come and, very rapidly, go.

The market is indeed cheaply and easily targeted. Neither Local
Swingers nor SDC charges for advertisement of parties, and the
swinging community invariably welcomes a new playground.

The swinging community, however, is a close one. Rumours and
news travel swiftly. Many swingers feel distinctly vulnerable. They
need to feel at ease, and soon complain of shiftless hosts, dirty skirting

boards, excessive heat or cold, and countless other factors which mar their relaxation. Above all, they need to know that they are secure and amongst fellows.

The would-be host and hostess, then, must invest heavily if they are to make the admittedly large profits to be gleaned this way. They must be house-proud and hospitable. And – a difficult act, this – they must be demonstrably swingers yet willing to forego swinging at their own parties. They must also accept that their house and grounds will be taken over by the enterprise.

Within weeks of our first swinging party, Lisa and I attended the first Secrets in a neo-Lutyens-style mansion in Devon's South Hams. There were then four downstairs rooms – a kitchen in which a basic buffet had been laid out; two large, thickly carpeted living-rooms, furnished in plush latter-day Parker-Knoll; and a conservatory with a hot-tub set into the floor – and four upstairs playrooms – a dark room furnished only with mattresses; a small private playroom; and two other rooms, one half-lit, one fully lit, in which our hosts' double-beds had been left and again the floors were covered with mattresses. The larger of these boasted a sex-swing. There were two loos, outside which there were always queues – and that was it.

It looked like what it was – the comfortable, modern country home of a sybaritic middle-aged couple – he a successful builder, she the manager of their considerable portfolio of rental properties. They had moved out all breakable ornaments and personal artefacts and had replaced any pictures with gentle, soft-core moody nudie posters.

Here, Chris – a crazy, energetic, white-haired and bespectacled player in his late fifties – and his lovely blonde wife Theresa, one of those perturbing, sexy creatures who are at once caring voluptuous matrons and sweet and sensuous glamour-girls, have resorted to a familiar subterfuge to deal with licensing laws. They sell raffle tickets which just incidentally entitle purchasers to a certain number of drinks from a bar.

The male bar staff are Chris's friends and employees. Stripped to the waist but for made-up bowties, they are allowed occasional twenty-minute breaks to mingle – as literally as they will – with the guests. They are the only single males allowed at Secrets.

Two years on, Secrets has a steaming swimming pool in the back garden, a second large jacuzzi, a steam-room, a sauna, a changing room, two additional loos, a garden playroom and a new room which houses the extensive buffet. It is hard to believe that this family home could now be anything but a swingers' venue.

Secrets is a success thanks to four principal factors. First, Chris and Theresa are genuine swingers, have explored the scene in depth and, like good chefs visiting rival restaurants, regularly attend other parties and clubs. Second, and almost paradoxically, they almost never play at their own parties. They are too busy being attentive, enthusiastic but unobtrusive hosts.

Third, they have the means to respond promptly to their guests' requirements and dissatisfactions. Finally – in part because they are swingers, in part because of their affability and solicitousness as hosts – they have a hardcore of regular, trustworthy guests who can be relied upon to attend and to get the party going.

As Richard and Janet, the hosts of another notable regular party at Radlett, north of London, say, 'We have seen a six-figure loss in the capital value of our home over the years. We do it because we are lucky enough to have a house like this and above all because we love it.'

Swingers, albeit wrongly, fear that tabloid journalists might be hovering to photograph their games or to reveal their identities (one reason that this fear is generally misguided is that I know many journalists of both genders who are swingers).

They fear that they might lose their jobs (they are wrong, unless they be politicians advocating the monogamous nuclear family or, perhaps, ministers of the Church. I would dearly love to see an employer humiliated by the courts for dismissing anyone for indulging a private, sexual preference with other consenting adults) or status.

They even fear, by what seems to be a conditioned paranoia, that they might be being set up or mocked for their passions.

Anyone, therefore, who is not a member of the subculture or who is felt to be exploiting them for money will very soon be discovered – and will fail.

Secrets and Radlett succeed because guests know that they are amongst their own kind. From the moment that they remove their coats and are greeted by their hosts, they can shed all pretences and play with confidence.

PART VII

1

SWINGING AND EMOTIONS

WHEN ALL THE PRACTICAL QUESTIONS are answered, the principal reason for hesitancy in joining the Lifestyle – whether as a swinger or merely as an observer and co-celebrant – is emotional uncertainty.

For most of us, this is virgin territory. We have inevitably fantasised about sex before an audience or with multiple partners, but we have broadly abided all our lives by the tenets of modesty and monogamy, serial or otherwise. We may like the notion of ourselves as porn stars, magnificent in rut and the objects of envy and desire, but we simply do not know how our bodies and minds will respond in such unfamiliar circumstances.

• • •

Modesty, of course, is not innate but the product of conditioning.

Although every child appears to inherit the problem at puberty and even the most experienced prostitute may still yelp and cover selected parts when surprised in the shower, specific perceptions and experiences of modesty vary so widely from culture to culture and from age to age – here men and women routinely expose their genitals whilst jealously covering their feet, here breasts are obsessively covered, there freely exposed – that it cannot be supposed to be an essential human trait.

It may, like lust awaiting a specific object or fear awaiting a cause, be a natural predisposition. But, if so, it is linked not to sexuality but to a more generalised body-awareness and sense of inadequacy or vulnerability within a hierarchy. It is born of fear and ignorance.

And no progeny of such monstrous parents can be good.

Many entirely proper and conventional people very readily shrug off clothes and modesty in mere minutes in health farms, changing rooms, at nudist beaches and colonies and in relationships of widely varying familiarity. So I have met no one who, despite initial fears, has found it hard to go naked at a swing-club or party where so many others are similarly exposed.

Curiously, given their often misplaced air of assurance, it is males who most frequently find themselves physiologically incapacitated in sexual performance by the lack of privacy.

This is not, as I have heard it suggested, because 'Women have less to do. They just have to lie there.' Not only is this evidently a misrepresentation of female functions, but repeated studies and experience have shown that women – once they are content that they are among friends – display far fewer inhibitions and fears than men and more readily give themselves up to the whole experience.

Men, however, whether through protectiveness, ignorance of their own sexuality in relation to that of other men (women seem naturally aware of the proper functions of their bodies without having to relate them to others), insecurity as to their size or proficiency or whatever factor, sometimes experience difficulties when first they undress in a crowd.

Again, couples are advised for this as for many other reasons to create their own space and to concentrate only on one another's pleasure – not merely initially but always. 'All the world loves a lover' in the Lifestyle as much as anywhere else, and the beauty of a couple plainly making love will, as an incidental benefit, attract the most sensitive, affectionate and confident couples.

2

SETTING LIMITS

OF COURSE, THE COUPLE NOW undressing to play will have determined in advance its own particular rules and limits.

It is as well here to stop well short of the limits of fantasy, which tend to be far-flung, and yet to be realistic.

One night at Secrets, Katy and I were playing beside a woman in her late thirties who, though a novice, was having the time of her life. We had met her earlier downstairs and she had told us of her nervousness and her delight at finding people in the Lifestyle 'so *normal*'.

Now she – call her Sharon – was alternately groaning like a blown kettle, yapping like a terrier and singing like a saw. Her cheeks and throat and the bibs of her little, bobbing breasts were puce. Her honey-coloured hair was painted in streaks across her face. She had entered that state of ecstatic erotic delirium where she was surfing all but blinded and powerless on breakers of sensation.

We had seen her on her back, being fucked by one man whilst she sucked another at her head. The woman lying on Sharon's other side stroked and fingered her. Then the man who had been fucking Sharon moved across to the second woman, and Sharon made the man at her head lie down. She straddled him, facing his feet, and her pelvis shuttled back and forth and swivelled round and round as she rode him.

Her head and mine were just inches apart. Her breath was hot on my lips. Her eyes focussed on mine. She smiled. She wrapped her arms around me, raised herself off the man and, pulling me down with her, lay down at Katy's left. They kissed.

Sharon looked up at me. She said, 'Go on. Fuck me. Please.'

I reached for a condom. Katy took me in her hand and guided me into Sharon. With the two girls still caressing one another and kissing beneath me, I did as I was told.

The writhing, grunting, gasping girl with her astonished, angry, blissful eyes gazed up at me. She looked unutterably beautiful, so I leaned down and kissed her. Her mouth was open, hot and welcoming as the rest of her.

The room seemed shaken by the sudden roar. 'No *kissing!*'

All heads turned.

A good-looking, muscular man was sitting on his heels, still sporting a vigorous erection but glowering, not ten feet from us. He had been there for a long while, but I had barely noticed him. Now I recognised him as Sharon's husband. His lips worked and his cheeks were flushed as his wife's.

He was not shouting at me, nor at any of the other people who had been playing with her. He was shouting at her. She had transgressed a very strange and wholly impractical rule. She had fucked, sucked and licked other men and women, but the two of them had evidently agreed that she would not kiss other men. Now, with my unwitting assistance, she had broken their rule.

Of course, they had got the whole thing wrong. Not only was their rule absurd, but she had 'got lucky' and had journeyed a long, long way from him, unaware, no doubt, that he had been reduced to the role of detached and presumably resentful spectator.

Maybe this denoted that they should not be playing. More probably – and perhaps these are the same things – it denoted that they should not be married.

So rules should be agreed with due regard to the frailties and yearnings of the human frame, in recognition that there will be many other opportunities to extend current limits and that any such extension must occur by spontaneous agreement before the event. There is a terrible tendency for newcomers to believe in the heat of the moment that this party or this encounter is the opportunity of a lifetime, and that sudden death must surely follow upon it.

Remember too that even the most experienced of couples has such limits, even if they are only 'no unprotected or anal sex with others'.

3

'LET THE GIRLS HAVE THEIR FUN'

SWINGING NOVICES TEND TO START OUT with things, rather than people, at the forefront of their minds.

They consciously and eagerly keep tally of the classic pornographic experiences and combinations which they enjoy. I certainly did – now two or three women gathered at my feet to share my genitals, now fucking a girl whilst she sucked another man or licked out another woman, now having my balls and arse licked by one woman as I fucked another or having one woman sit on my face whilst another rode my cock, now engaging in double penetration and so on.

Within a couple of months, all these – though every bit as pleasurable as I had conjectured (a rarity in itself) – were familiar pleasures with manifold variations rather than accomplishments. In true Platonic style, I could then move on to concentrate on the people in all their miraculous sameness and their multifarious, intoxicating differences.

Although less liable than men to separate acts from people and to make lists, women too as they enter the Lifestyle tend to invest particular acts with the daunting status of obstacles to be surmounted – the first blow-job, the first pussy, the first fuck, the first spit-roast and so on.

It is a very foolish swing-partner who attempts to expedite this course. Some people will plunge straight into the depths of orgiastic sex. Others must feel their way, step by step, analysing each new attainment and ensuring that the riverbed is secure and contains no stinging surprises.

Oh, and one last golden rule for male swingers: LET THE GIRLS HAVE THEIR FUN.

Many a swinging meet and many a successful encounter at an orgy will start with the women playing together, kissing, caressing, joking, lapping, humming and purring for what may seem hours.

Let it happen. Go and make a drink for them. Chat amongst yourselves about movies or music or, if you must, traffic, football or whatever ordinary men talk about. Occasionally and unobtrusively murmur words of appreciation of the view and declare your desires. Maybe kneel beside them and kiss your partner, but do not intrude.

Of course, they may immediately want the cock in the cocktail, but often it will be an hour or more before they have had enough of one another – and, of course, of teasing you.

But face it. Their stamina exceeds yours, and, by the time that they have enjoyed this much 'foreplay' – and, of course, teasing you – and feel the need for male hands, male lips and cock, your welcome is assured and your patience will be rewarded many times over. Interfere, however, in what may be for them a rare treat, and introduce a different time-scale – an urgent jingle in the midst of an adagio – and you run the risk of being seriously irritating.

Unless they hate you very much, the women have not forgotten you as they play. You are just the second (the *entrée?*) course.

4

JEALOUSY

JEALOUSY IS A PECULIARLY hideous passion, and swingers are no less vulnerable to it than anyone else.

Expect it. Expect the twinges or jolts as you watch your partner kissing or caressing another, and appreciate that he or she will experience similar shocks as you first play with others.

Make the effort, therefore, to reassure him, to take his hand, to kiss him, to smile at him and to feel and express pride and awe at his beauty as he plays. Become too engrossed in your own pleasure and you run the risk of losing not only your future in the Lifestyle but your partner into the bargain.

For all that initial apprehensiveness, swingers routinely have sex as couples with others and declare that, far from afflicting them with the pathological torment which has destroyed so many lives, it brings them closer and consolidates the bonds between them.

This is not because swingers are freaks. They know jealousy. Many of them, although members of the Lifestyle for many years, declare that they are still susceptible to it in their everyday dealings. When swinging, however, it never crosses their minds or adversely affects their pleasure or their love for one another.

How does this work?

Nothing better illustrates the fact that sexual jealousy is seldom if ever proportionate to its cause.

A simple and commonplace sexual act, which might signify no more than passing lust, is transformed in the mind of the sufferer into an act of personal violence to him or her, an act of sacrilege and iconoclasm which violates his or her most sacred beliefs and ideals, a rejection of any love, friendship or undertaking which precedes that moment.

In this sense, it is an emotion founded upon surreal (and pathetically self-important) imaginings, because few if any sexual acts are, or represent, all or any of these things. They may be motivated by loneliness, lust, pity, rebelliousness, drunkenness or indeed vindictiveness. If the transgressor returns to the initial relationship hoping that it can still be maintained, however, it is clear that these were transitory aberrations only (though the aggrieved partner may reasonably conclude, particularly where there is deceit, that he or she may 'on form' be likely to transgress again and so may not share the partner's views of fidelity's importance).

A rational man or woman could make this appraisal. Jealousy, however, is the ultimate self-feeding monster. This is its hellish nature. It conceives and elaborates its own causes. It complains of wounds which it then proceeds to probe, extend and liberally season. It deliberately explores in detail and with relish what it should – in all reason – shy from, and, where there is no such detail, supplies it.

It does not allow that the transgressors may lead normal lives, have normal worries and perform commonplace functions. They must spend every waking moment in disgusting, inventive, skilful, mocking sex.

A huge part of sexual jealousy is founded upon such paranoiac speculation, and the remainder, surely, upon a sense of betrayal – the sense that something thought to be exclusive has proved, without the consent of one of the parties, to be inclusive, the thoughts of intimacies and endearments, gifts, confidences and pledges which may have been shared (and that 'may' is crucial, again allowing truly infinite possibilities) to the exclusion – the treacherous exclusion – of the jealous one.

'Doubt is the chief torture of the jealous man who remains sane,' writes Gonzales-Crussi in 'On the Nature of Things Erotic'. 'True jealousy never stems from the absolute certainty that one is deceived, but from suspecting the possibility of deceit. "Does she love someone else?" "Is she the one I thought she was …?"

For swingers (to whom the answers to the above questions are an undoubting 'No' and a joyous 'Yes') the astounding – though, on consideration, obvious – discovery is that, where there is no room for speculation and demonstrably no betrayal of the core relationship, sex itself is no cause for jealousy at all. When shared with a partner in clearly finite, delimited circumstances, sex is neither an act of commitment nor a warrant of exclusivity, but a delightful game only. An actor's husband will not be jealous of her love scenes on stage. If he is not a fellow actor, however, he might well be tormented by worries as to just what is going on in rehearsals in his absence.

Those initial twinges felt by new swingers are of uncertainty. Remove the uncertainty and jealousy is gone.

'What always gets me is how stunningly beautiful she is when she's playing,' says Michael, of Fiona – his wife of 14 years. 'She's happy and stunning and filled up and glowing. I just feel so fucking proud of her. I mean, you never really get to see someone when you're fucking or eating them, so you never realise till you get to watch them just how gorgeous and sexy and amazing they are.

'And afterwards, when we get home, there's my own megastar in bed with me, just with me, and it's heaven. And when I look at her –

I don't know, doing the kids or dolled up for some business thing – I just think, "Hey. Look at my sexy superstar ..."'

'It's just a huge turn-on to see him looking so happy and to watch the girlies he's playing with,' agrees Fiona, of Michael. 'And I swear I can be in a pile of bodies and he touches me and I know immediately who it is. It just sort of shudders through me. If he ever cheated on me – well, why would he? – I'd rip his balls off, and I know it would tear him apart if I ever tried to deceive him. But, like I say, why would we? It would make no sense.'

'There really is almost nothing else that makes us feel so close,' says Nicki, of her relationship with Marcus. 'I mean, this is what sex is meant to do but so seldom does – an exclusive, shared thing which reveals the innermost you, vulnerable ... powerful ... playing out intimate fantasies ... fully alive – naked in every way. And this lovely, passionate human being is all mine, and is sharing all of who he is with me, and encouraging me to be me and loving me for it. You beat that.'

Again and again, you will hear the same testimony from swingers.

Playing together with others is for them what sex between two people (in the relationship's early days, at least) used to be – a cumulatively exclusive revelation, a sharing of otherwise concealed impulses, yearnings and vulnerabilities, a conjuring of beloved and essential monsters from darkness into the light of a beloved's gaze, in hope that he will hug them to him and match them, creature for creature, and that these long-imprisoned creatures will greet one another as kin and rejoice in their liberty and romp with one another like children.

Copulation, for better or for worse, has become, in itself, a commonplace – or, it might be argued, has resumed its proper status (again I stress that I do not dispute its ability to be transfigured, as can a commonplace leaf or landscape, into a token of the divine) after a century of being elevated to quasi-sacred status.

Few of us now are terrified that we might be mocked for failing to function normally, that we might become pregnant without our volition, or that our hearts might be stolen and sold off cheap in the mere process of fucking.

It is not fucking which has changed. It is the often unwanted commitments which once it entailed and the fears which once attended it, which have now been removed. To return to Lisa's gastronomic metaphor, when we are no longer afraid of poisoning or driven by fear of starvation, it is the feast or the shared visit to a special restaurant rather than the home-cooked meal which becomes the exciting, special shared experience.

And so, for swingers, it is the vicarious enjoyment of a partner's pleasure (not to mention sharing the food off the other's plate – always more delicious than one's own) which creates the peculiar bond.

Jealousy is not extinct in them. Deception or secrecy would hurt and anger them as much as more conventionally monogamous couples, but deception and secrecy are all but unknown to swingers, who count themselves monogamous despite the many people with whom they may play.

'Play is fantasy,' says Donna, 37 – a gorgeous, blonde, multi-orgasmic sports instructor from Bridgwater – who, with her charming husband Dave, 45, is one of the most respected swingers in southern Britain, 'and there's not a monogamous person in the world who doesn't have fantasy sex with people other than their partners.

'But non-swingers mix the two things up and go off in their own heads when they're fucking. We have our fantasy sex together and with other people, and when we have real sex alone together, we're into one another more than ever before, and it's just him and me, being real and wanting to be together, not using one another while we think of other people. I've never been unfaithful to David in reality or in my mind since we started playing.'

Between them, these two have had sex with hundreds of people over the past ten years, yet neither has ever been unfaithful to one another in that time, and both regard infidelity as shameful and just cause for the breakdown of a marriage.

Almost all swingers scorn the notion of the 'open marriage' on empirical grounds. 'We've seen a few attempts, but we've never known such a thing to work in the long-term,' says Donna. 'Another relationship creates a distance between you – all that "Did I say that to him, or him? Did I do that with him, or him?" All that suspicion that she may be better than you, or that he may be doing more for her than for you. You can't live with that. Well, not if your primary relationship is a loving one.'

'Don't make out you've never been jealous though,' Dave teases.

'Mm, yes, there've been a couple of women I thought he seemed to be paying too much attention to,' admits Donna, 'but we in the Lifestyle have a simple solution to that.'

She smiles and demonstrates that Bonobosexual politics are alive and well in human relationships.

'I fuck them,' she says simply. 'Make them mine as well. Bingo. Threat gone.'

5

KAMIKAZE SPERM

TO MANY, THE EMOTIONS OF swingers are alien and incomprehensible. It seems, however, that, when conditioned responses are erased, there are sound physiological reasons for their pleasures and penchants.

In common with most subcultures which have discovered something marvellous to them yet inexplicable to others, swingers cling to whatever scientific validation they can find.

The findings of Robin Baker of Manchester University, who, in 1996, published *Sperm Wars: The Science of Sex,*[1] are therefore more widely known and quoted by swingers than might be expected of a serious study by an evolutionary biologist.

Baker and his colleague Mark Bellis analysed the ejaculate found in the condoms of their cohabiting students. They made a startling discovery. When a man suspects or knows his woman to have had sex with another man, he manufactures a vastly increased number of sperm. They further discovered that less than one-tenth of these

[1]Robin Baker and Mark Bellis, *The Science of Sex*, New York: Basic Books, 1996

sperm are actually programmed to fertilise the ovum. The remainder are 'kamikaze sperm', whose sole function is to destroy any rivals injected by another male and to make straight the way for their champions.

This, coupled with the innumerable studies which have shown that women – though sometimes satisfied – are genetically programmed to be sexually insatiable and to seek variety in their sexual partners, certainly explains much of the extraordinary pleasure reported by both genders in swinging and in that special 'last dance' retained for partners.

Remove outmoded social conditioning, insecure proprietary claims and, above all, the ignorance upon which jealousy depends for its existence (nowhere is '*tout comprendre, c'est tout pardonner*' truer), and the manifold pleasures of multiple sexual partners and mass-production of kamikaze sperm can be enjoyed within a loving, emotionally exclusive relationship.

Again, on much the same principle as that which dictates that producers of peanuts must print a warning on the packet declaring that 'This product may contain nuts', I stress that not everyone is capable of shrugging off such conditioning.

All would-be swingers should start out with extensive discussion and visualisation and should dip their toes in the deep pool of the Lifestyle very, very cautiously, being prepared – if that be all that is practicable – to enjoy the novel sensations of wet toes, to add it to the sum total of experiences binding a couple together and to proceed no further.

6

'TONGUES, OR HE'LL SUSPECT!'

SWINGERS MAY OVERCOME JEALOUSY and strive for emotional clarity and order, but they are as subject as anyone else to the confusions caused by overwhelming needs.

With secure established couples, such needs are rare. It is, as ever, where definitions become blurred and categories confused that there is a threat.

I fell foul of such confusion.

• • •

'For God's sake, talk about fucking!'

On the monitor, Sally glanced nervously over her shoulder. Her husband had returned earlier than expected.

She had heard his cry of greeting and his footfalls on the stairs up to the attic where they kept their computers. She and I been talking on webcam and Messenger about her dogs.

This was altogether too intimate.

I tapped in the words as fast as I could: 'I can't wait to feel your pussy bobbing before my face again, to spank you till your arse is bright pink, to kiss you as I come deep inside you, then to feel you pulsing around me as we subside ...'

She was looking up now, talking to the dark man who stood over her, clutching a steaming mug. She nodded a couple of times. He gestured towards the screen. She talked some more.

'...I keep thinking of how you ate that little blonde thing as we were fucking on Wednesday,' I wrote, 'and how you both sucked me afterwards. We must do that again, *now,* and this time I'll come in both your mouths ...'

She was still nodding as she turned back to the screen. She had obviously minimised our conversation window. Now she restored it. She read this gibberish and grinned broadly. She indicated the screen. Her husband leaned forward to read. He waved at me.

She typed, 'Clay says hi and how come we get all the fun?'

I grinned and waved back. In the topsy-turvy, Saturnalian world of swinging, I had proved our innocence.

Talk of dogs was incriminating. Talk of sex was just fine.

On another occasion, when I had been lying atop Sally at Secrets, she had pinched my buttock and gasped in my ear, 'Tongues, or he'll suspect!' I had been kissing her, it seemed, on her brow, her nose, her lips, her throat with my lips closed. This was a breach of protocol.

We were meant to be swinging. Instead, it was plain, we had slipped into an affair.

7

HOTWIFE

FOR THREE MONTHS AFTER Lisa's departure, I had been continuing my researches with a series of transitory partners from all over the country. I was desperate for a regular swing-partner when first I met Sally through SDC, where she not only had a couple's profile with her husband, but – with his encouragement – a profile as a single female.

She turned up at my cottage in a Mazda glass slipper one sunny June evening. She wore a swirly black dress ticked with white. Her hair was short and blonde. She was very slim. I later learned that she ran ten miles twice a week, was in training for a marathon and was a regular kick-boxer. Her legs were lovely.

She had one of those faces which, when animated, seemed to light up the entire room but, when allowed to relax, often seemed punctured and expressive of all the weariness and grief in the world. It challenged you to make it happy. It right royally rewarded success.

That first evening, after she had had just one glass of wine, we moved into the bedroom, and had lovely, loving, playful and very vigorous sex. Breaking her own rules, Sally rang her husband to ask if she might spend the night with me. He assented. She told me, 'I'll have to pay. I go back smelling of you tomorrow, he'll jump on me straight away.'

For six months, still with her husband's consent – if not his entire approval – Sally had attended parties with me in Bristol, London, Birmingham, Newport and Leicester. She had organised and attended meets with me and declared her eagerness to explore further afield.

She was an ardent, sensuous and adventurous lover. Aside from our swinging nights, she spent every Wednesday night with me. We set up our own profile on swingers' sites. It was only logical to give her a couple of drawers and a section of the wardrobe in which to store her play clothes …

● ● ●

Sally was what is known in the Lifestyle as a 'hotwife'.

Women whose sexual appetites exceed their partners' are many, but some of these are fortunate enough to have partners who – despite their own relative inactivity – derive pleasure from their wives' or girlfriends' adventures.

Hotwives in stable relationships are a huge social asset. Hotwives like Sally are dangerous.

Her marriage was obviously foundering. She often treated Clay with disdain, then invariably regretted it. She had been reared in a military family, had married young, joined the Navy and had risen to the rank of Chief Petty Officer. Her first marriage – after a brief, dis-astrous foray into vanilla-style, messy extempore swinging – had broken down. She had immediately married Clay – a colleague who fantasised about swinging and plainly welcomed what many would consider humiliation at Sally's hands.

All her life, then, she had been protected and confined by orderly institutions. Two years ago, she had left the Navy. She now had her own small property-finding business. She was 41 and she wanted to try freedom.

I had thought that we could help one another and that I could afford her emotional support through a difficult transitional period – maybe even help her to deal with her frustrations and enable her to remain with Clay, who seemed to me a nice, if dull, guy.

From the moment when she wrote, 'For God's sake talk about fucking!' I realised that this was, for her, no longer play. We were involved in deceit.

We discussed it. There were tears. We agreed that we must take a break.

Sally even organised the succession as a parting gift. She arranged to attend Secrets one night with Clay, which meant that I needed another partner for the night. She had come across – sorry, she had met – 24-year-old Katy, who had also been in the Navy, and reckoned that we would get on.

Katy came over to my place one afternoon. She is a Yorkshire girl. We sat in the sunshine and discussed the Lyke Wake walk, the Tredentine Mass and anal sex. We then went to bed. It was good.

Two days later, we went to Secrets. Clay drove us there. Sally sat beside him in the passenger seat. Katy sucked my cock in the back seat, and I wound Sally up by feeding her the taste of Katy on my fingers.

This may have been valedictory, but Sally and I were friends and confused. A strange female battle for precedence took place that night. Katy, Sally and I played together from 9.30pm until 2.30 am. At one stage, we spent two full hours in the large playroom with the two girls licking one another to orgasm again and again whilst I fucked them, moving from one end of their entwined bodies to the other. When at last we decided to stagger downstairs for a drink, we realised that we had attracted an audience. Eight couples standing around us actually broke into applause. We blushed.

Downstairs, we resumed on the canopied bed. Now the girls took turns with me, and their caresses for one another were rougher. At one stage, Katy was riding me as I lay on my back. Sally, who had been lying beside me kissing me, announced, 'I want that cock.' She knelt up, grabbed a double handful of Katy's abundant auburn hair, pulled her head back, kissed her and spat into her mouth. 'RHIP,' she said. 'Off.' She pushed Katy off me and sank onto me herself.

'What was that about?' I asked Katy later.

'"Rank Has Its Privileges",' Katy explained. 'I was a rating. She was a Chief – though she never went to sea, so it doesn't really count. I can't believe she pulled rank on me, the bitch!'

Sally was handing me on, but she needed to establish her precedence.

Three weeks later, it was my birthday. Katy had been visiting me often from her home in Bournemouth, but Sally had decided that the event was still hers to control. She had organised a party for six couples at my cottage on the Saturday, but, the night before that, she officially gave me Katy.

Katy had been sworn to secrecy, but had told me nonetheless, so I had to feign surprise when Sally turned up, arm-in-arm with the younger girl. 'Birthday present one,' she said, pushing Katy into my arms. 'I've got my period, but I want you two to play.'

So we did.

It was a strange scene. Katy and I obediently played. Sally drank champagne and watched approving. Sometimes she came over and kissed us, frigged Katy or sucked me, but she spent most of the night sitting crosslegged on the bedside or in the armchair and murmuring to us as we fucked. When at last I came, it was in Katy's mouth – the one forbidden, exclusive intimacy.

Katy did not swallow. She leaped off the bed, strode over to Sally, pulled her head back and spat fiercely into her mouth before kissing her.

Honours, I supposed, were even.

The following week, Katy took over as my partner.

8

THE DANGER OF REALITY

THE HARSH FACT WHICH, in my eagerness, I had neglected to observe was that Sally and I had not, on those Wednesday nights alone, just been swinging any more.

Yes, I had met her through a swinging site and she and Clay had had a few swinging meets together, and yes, she and I had played together as a couple with many other people.

Her status as a married female playing solo, however, albeit with Clay's encouragement, was a fake. He had encouraged her because he enjoyed the thought of her with others, but also because he had held onto some vague, vain hope that they might thus preserve the status quo. In fact, she was irrevocably on the move and seeking a wagon to which to hitch her star. Unlike all other intentions in the Lifestyle, none of these was explicit or openly shared.

Dangers of such emotional confusion are present in all milieux. The same situation might as well have arisen had Sally and I been low-handicap golfers and Clay an unambitious, admiring and gener-

ous plodder, or we playing the leads in an amateur theatrical production whilst he was an ASM.

The fact that swingers' hobby involves sex makes the danger less,
not greater, in that their *confrères* and *soeurs* are explicitly committed
to sex as an expression of desire and friendship freely shared – not
withheld as an ultimate prize – and to emotional bonds as inviolable
and dissociated from physical pleasure.

Where single players are involved, however, and particularly
where couples separate to pursue their own ends, swinging runs a
high risk of ceasing to be play.

All our single swinger friends play with couples and other singles,
as did I throughout that period. But even where the couple consists
of a woman who plays and her partner is to all intents and purposes a
spectator, it is essential that they arrive and leave together and that
singles genuinely are singles.

All else places swingers at risk of precisely the emotional mess
which they are at such pains, by their lifestyle choice, to avoid.

9

GIVING UP SWINGING

SALLY DID LEAVE HER HUSBAND – and swinging. A month after we split, she moved to Cheltenham to be near her family. She rented a little country cottage. For a while, she remained on the site as a single female. Then she fell in love. For now at least, she is no longer a player. She elects, however, to live alone.

'Looking back, I'm really glad that happened, though it hurt like hell at the time. One of us had to realise what was happening and stop it,' she admits now.

'Clay had given me a taste for swinging. He enjoyed the fantasy and he liked watching me, and I suppose we both hoped it might bring us back together. But I just loved it. I realised what I'd been missing all that time. I felt that I'd been cheated all my life up till then. And I discovered girls, which is just fantastic. Our marriage was already on the rocks, and here was this new group of really happy, together people who made me welcome and gave me friendship and the best sex ever.

'So I knew I wanted out. I think I'd always known I wanted out, but I was really scared. I didn't know anything except being in a relationship with a man. The idea of being on my own was intoxicating but terrifying, so then I met you, and you were in the Lifestyle and wanted independence which made you really attractive, and what do I do when I find something attractive and independent? Try to catch it of course. Keep it for myself. Victorian naturalist. Hey, look, how beautiful. That bird is flying so high. I know, let's shoot it and stuff it and that way I can keep it. Derrr. And I didn't even realise that was what I was doing till you told me ...

'Will I stay out of the Lifestyle now? I don't know. I really miss it. I miss my friends. I miss the thrill every week of dressing up and not knowing what might happen. I miss the variety. If George ever wanted to do it, I'd be back like a shot, but he's not comfortable with it, and he's what matters.

'It really is very hard to think I might never be part of it again. You should warn people about that. It's like being a sportsman, I think. The excitement, the companionship, the wind-in-your-hair, fuck-it-all fun of it all ... It's hard to replace that.'

Sally's departure from the Lifestyle highlights another emotional problem confronted by swingers. Just how easy is it to dismount from this tiger? It is certainly an addictive pastime, offering to its members freedom, excitement, self-esteem and an international society. It might be compared to active participation in a high-risk sport, and it is well-known that sportsmen and women find it hard to adjust to a life without the camaraderie and stimulus afforded by their game, and often resort to substitutes such as gambling and drink.

I have, however, known many individuals and couples who have given up swinging, though none who has renounced it for good. They have only, like Sally, 'taken a break' on a 'wait and see' basis. This is probably just the commonsense caution practised by alcoholics or drug addicts who vow sobriety 'one day at a time'.

There are many good reasons – but only nebulous consolations –

for giving up drink or drugs. There are only two reasons (age and injury) – and no consolations at all – for giving up sport or battle. The only reasons for renouncing swinging (aside from the weariness of age, which also blessedly diminishes desire) are pregnancy, a sudden affliction of religious belief, or a similar conversion to passionate love for a non-swinger. These are sufficiently immediate and engrossing to make such a transition easy.

I have encountered swinging nerds – people to whom swinging is a substitute for married life, sport and all other leisure activities. Their entire lives are taken up with planning for swinging, and with net and webcam conversations with a view to meetings. For these, giving up swinging must be nigh impossible. Their lives would be empty without it. I suspect that their lives are empty with it.

For most of us, however, swinging is an occasional entertainment and stimulus. I realise that any book that takes as its subject a specific leisure activity – be it theatre, rock-climbing, stamp-collecting or swinging – must give the impression that it is a constant preoccupation or even an obsession. In fact, my partners and I have averaged perhaps two orgies and a couple of meets a month, and, after the initial rush, have seldom spent more than two hours a week in chatting to potential partners online or on the telephone.

Despite the multiplicity of partners – and, of course, the duration of sex at parties, where it is not uncommon to play more or less continually for five or six hours – I doubt that we had much more sex as swingers than we would have had as a normal, active couple in the first, lustful days of an affair. It was just that those first, lustful days endured for as long as we were together.

We worked, we kept houses and livestock and we conducted social lives aside from swinging. Swinging was a diversion, something to look forward to and back on. When – as occasionally happened – we went a couple of months without an orgy, due to work or family commitments, it caused no great restlessness or distress.

If, however, one of us had suddenly announced that he or she intended to give up swinging, I suspect that the tensions would have been great and that the entire relationship might have foundered. But then, I suspect that a couple for whom golf or yachting were central to their social and leisure lives might have found a unilateral renunciation of that pastime equally difficult to bear. Luckily, this was never put to the test.

When this book and my recovery probation period are done, I may no longer dutifully accept every invitation nor quite so avidly tour the country in search of new experience, but I will inevitably still have friends in the Lifestyle. I will visit them and they me, and I certainly cannot see myself turning aloof and censorious should they start to play or suggest a visit to a party.

Occasionally there will be an irresistibly interesting party. Occasionally swinging will need a champion and, if I can be of any service, I will step up to the mark. Already, perhaps for no better reason than that I am literate and well-spoken, I am asked by the curious to hold their metaphorical hands as they make their own explorations of the scene or to offer them some guidance when they are troubled. Again, I can see no reason for refusing.

I suspect that this is how most swingers 'give up'. Like athletes, they retain their contacts and continue to turn out for occasional events and to help their successors in the field. There is no wrench. It remains an important but increasingly peripheral part of their lives.

A month will pass without swinging, then, one day, six months, and they notice it, and notice that they have not missed it, and shrug, perhaps a little surprised. They would never classify themselves as 'ex-swingers', since that would imply a renunciation of the entire Lifestyle.

It is altogether too exciting, agreeable, kindly and entertaining, and its philosophy too congenial, for that.

PART VIII

1

ANTECEDENTS AND INFLUENCES

SEX STARTED IN 1929.

It has seldom been observed – and seems incredible to many – that the most powerful marketing tool in the world, the touchstone of modern morality, the bugbear of all puritans, a term which denotes a million practices, pleasures and pains, did not even exist a century ago.

It has a great deal to answer for, especially for something whose meaning is as yet undefined.

I have used the word as a convenient shorthand throughout this book, but I for one have little idea what it means.

Is masturbation sex? Can an infant then 'have sex with' a rocking-horse? Is caressing one's own nipples sex? And, if not, is caressing the nipples of another?

At what point do kissing or heavy petting become sex? Is digital penetration of a pussy or arse sex? If so, are proctologists and gynae-cologists professional sex workers? Should a woman feel guilty because she experiences pleasures related to the sexual when breast-feeding? What sort of unholy mess has this extraordinary word made of our perception of ourselves and our natural functions?

Or must we accept that pernicious eighteenth- and nineteenth-century notion that the only real sex is defined by male penetration and internal ejaculation, and that all else is mere perversion, preparatory to, or unnaturally replacing, 'the real thing'?

If that be the case, then the history of sex is straightforward. For many millennia, penises have entered the necks of wombs and squirted out semen. And cervices (when female orgasm has been permitted) have swooped down to suck up that semen. Sometimes this has resulted in babies. End of story.

But of course that is not the nature of sex but merely the mechanics of conception, which can be replicated *in vitro* or with a turkey-baster.

Before 1929 when, characteristically, DH Lawrence first used this almost meaningless term, your 'sex' was your gender or the defining organ or organs of your gender. It was not a broad, all-encompassing category of activities which could be approved, desired or deplored.

You might feel an urgent longing to eat a specific pussy, suck a specific cock, fuck, be fucked or simply have an orgasm, but you could not 'feel like sex' or 'want sex', nor was it ever argued that bondage, say, spanking or oral intercourse were 'sex' and so must be restricted to a particular social contract.

The practice of 'bundling', whereby courting couples, partially clothed and on occasion separated by a 'bundling board', would share a bed with the full approval of their parents, is characteristic of former ages which acknowledged the joys of mutual gratification without (it was hoped) penetration.

Though clerics grumbled about the custom, bundling persisted in rural Celtic areas of Europe and in North America until the late nineteenth century and beyond. Pregnancies might and did result and the errant couple was then expected to marry, but it is clear that bundling existed precisely to enable intimacy and sexual play.

Such relative personal liberalism within a rigidly structured soci-ety contrasts instructively with contemporary 'sex-consciousness', which serves to proscribe adult proximity to children and even two male friends sharing a bed (though phallocentricity here inadver-tently gives women a degree of licence here. After all, they cannot possibly have sex.).

We owe much of this to Lawrence's silly, lazy neologism.

2

ORGIES AS SEASONAL CONTRACEPTION?

THE HISTORY OF GROUP SEX IS no doubt as long as that of human coupling.

Certainly public sex is or was the norm for humans, as for other species. When life was 'nasty, brutish and short', a couple's withdrawal from the family or tribe for something as commonplace as sexual intercourse would have been downright daft.

The haystack, so beloved of film directors as a scene of rumpy pumpy, may indeed have been the place where most of our ancestors were conceived, though the warmth of the communal dung heap probably gives it prior claims.

Of course, public sex does not denote group sex, nor can we suppose – for all human females' constant receptivity and probable promiscuity – that they will have been, as many have surmised, indiscriminately available or constantly pregnant. Monogamy (or, more probably, polygyny) and tribalism will have afforded some protection from ceaseless rape by young males, but there was surely an additional restraint.

In paleolithic times, mankind appears to have been divided into hunters and hunter-gatherers. Whilst the hunters would have migrated in pursuit of their prey over vast distances every year, the hunter-gatherers dwelled in caves and moved to the hills in summer to make the most of the game and fresh pastures. Long before they were dependent on animal husbandry or the growth of crops, then, humans must have been aware of seasons and structured their lives about them.

Whether in the ice-ages or in more temperate ages, it must also have been clear that there were provident times at which to travel and at which to breed.

A woman can both conceive and give birth just once in a calendar year. With lactational amenorrhea, she can then extend the period during which she can enjoy sex without risk of conception for several years. We need not suppose that children were born at random dates throughout the year and that those born at certain seasons simply died of malnutrition or were killed as encumbrances to the tribe. Paleolithic and neolithic man and woman were perfectly capable of maximising their efficiency in breeding and the chances of their offspring's survival by copulating at the most propitious time.

Avebury in Wiltshire, with its giant stone circles and avenues, its prodigious ditches and, perhaps most remarkable of all, the gigantic manmade tumulus of Silbury Hill, is the greatest construct ever created by human endeavour. It is of course a neolithic complex, built at a time when humans were farmers and kept domestic animals and so were well aware of gestation periods.

Avebury stands on the Ridgeway, the appositely named, elevated road which once stretched right across southern England from Dorset to Norfolk. In the days when Avebury was perhaps the greatest centre of civilisation in Western Europe, that road was the sole means of travel which did not mean battling through bog and dense forest peopled with savage beasts and outlaws.

I have heard many hypotheses as to the purpose of Avebury, most of them to do with ley-lines, the positions of the stars and other New

Age preoccupations. It was a local stonemason, however, the twenty-third of that calling in direct line, who gave me the first account which ever made sense.

'What my family always said – nowadays people say "Was it religious?" or "Was it political?", which are questions which make sense to us who've separated everything into categories ... Wouldn't have meant anything to the folks that built this place – was that once a year, when it was safe to travel, people came here from all over the country to trade, make alliances, perform religious rites and find mates.

'And there were permanent priests here, and the circles were actually conference halls – maybe even where the story of Arthur's Round Table came from centuries later. So each chieftain would have a protective stone when he entered the circle unarmed, maybe with their own people armed behind the stone – and Lord knows what was in the centre. Wouldn't surprise me if it was a big pole.

'Round here we still call Silbury Hill "the hill of the golden nights", because it's obviously a big busting fertility thing and all the women who'd been bought or wooed or traded or whatever went up there with the men and they had a huge orgy in the hope that there'd be a baby in December or January, because that'd leave the mother fit for sowing and for harvest this year and next and the child fit for travelling at the beginning of next summer.'

The notion of seasonal orgies as, effectively, contraceptives for the rest of the year and means to the avoidance of incest (or, at least, of its baleful consequences) is an extraordinary but persuasive one.

Of course, it may be that humans merely responded instinctively to the rising sap and reflorescence of spring as supposed by the poets and songwriters, but folk tradition outlives records, and the persistent conventions of Fasching, carnival, the Feast of Fools, the Maypole and the like – always in late spring, overtly sexual and dedicated to the overthrowing of established status, usually by means of masks – give credence to my informant's explanation.

We have endlessly been told since the nineteenth century of 'fertility rites' in which, it seems, people danced around sexual symbols or paid cult to gods and goddesses of regeneration in hope of good harvests.

This is bowdlerised anthropology. Do we really still believe that they did so without fucking, or that these rites were not intended to make their fucking propitious rather than the other way round? If so, look at the accounts of Maypole dancing in the sixteenth century, at which two-thirds of the females were said to be 'defiled' – or, for that matter, attend Carnival in Venice or Rio to this day.

It would certainly have made sense for people to hold an orgy at the spring festivals, and for female sex to have been polyandrous at those times in order to enhance prospects of conception.

Much has been made by evolutionary biologists and anthropologists of the fact that primitive and isolated peoples have been found who appear unaware of the connection between coitus and childbirth. I have yet to find one such instance which is convincing.

It is traditional – and in keeping with the racism of colonialism – that we make our ancestors out to be idiots and so aggrandising ourselves. So children are brought up to this day to believe that, until Columbus, everyone believed the world to be flat. This is demonstrable nonsense.

It *is* barely possible that earlier nomadic hunter-gatherers failed to make the connection between sex and childbirth. It is certain that conception was widely associated with other factors, such as the intervention of the gods, the sun, the moon (aptly), amulets, charms and ceremonies. It has been, and still is, in our own societies today.

It may be that people were unaware that one single emission of semen in the vagina was sufficient to do the entire job. It is not feasible, however, to suppose that a hugely sophisticated, agrarian society of animal husbandmen and crop-growers such as that of our Neolithic ancestors, was unaware that fornication was linked to birth.

3

THE PERSISTENCE OF ORGIES

DESPITE THE FACT THAT MOST early history was written by men with political axes to grind or by clerics, it is clear that there were orgies in Sumeria and in Babylon, in ancient Greece and Rome and in all ancient civilisations. Most of these – or those of which we have records – were nominally associated with religious observance, but then, in pantheistic societies, they would have been.

We who are reared in monotheistic tradition see the Lesbian festival of Aphrodite Asonia, say, held annually in Thessaly, or the Bacchanalia which swept third-century BC Italy, either as religious festivals abused or as orgies claiming divine sanction.

To the pagan mind, such distinctions were meaningless. I am confident that those who attended these festivals did so with the same excited anticipation as that with which today's swingers prepare for parties. The very strange distinction between the physical and the spiritual had not at this point been made.

Orgies have consistently continued throughout history, though those most frequently acknowledged by Western chroniclers were of the organised, seasonal, parareligious variety which survived in rural areas into the nineteenth century.

From the sixteenth and seventeenth centuries onward, the clerical monopoly on the written word had been broken (though Christian despite of the flesh by now prevailed throughout the Western world) and metropolitan society was well-established and organised. If the surviving poets, diarists and novelists – most of them concerned for their social reputations – represent one-tenth of the truth, group sex appears to have been widespread, both in the court and in the brothel.

How closely can we relate such activities – private and privileged on the one hand and public and democratic on the other – to modern swinging? Alas for apologists, barely at all.

4

DOLLYMOPS AND MIDINETTES

THE SURVIVAL OF ORGIASTIC FESTIVALS and the tendency of the most privileged urban people – kings, queens, their courts and, more recently, film stars and rock stars – to resort to such diversions whenever practical may be seen as suggestive of an enduring predisposition.

Marriage, however, has meant very different things to different ages. The 'respectable' women (as distinct from those born privileged) of whom we retain records are rarely to be found *in flagrante*. This may be because low-sexed, highly conditioned women won social and economic success whilst their more wanton sisters were a drug on the social and marital markets. It may be that chroniclers simply turned a blind eye to the exceptions.

Either way, the Christian jackboot never succeeded in trampling insatiable female sexuality to death. We need only look to case-studies of those deemed insane or possessed – the accounts of mass self-flagellation throughout mediaeval Europe and the wild evidence in the witch-trials of the fifteenth and sixteenth centuries – to recognise that neither knowledge of 'sexual' excesses, nor the wildest 'sexual' fantasies and desires, ever abated.

The more I studied the history of sexualities and the more I observed swingers, the more I recognised that both fly in the face of the most pervasive of stereotypes – that of the female as 'naturally' monogamous.

Where conception is possible, the female's potential biological investment is obviously far greater than the male's, and she quite reasonably prefers to bet on high cards. Devotion is a king and wealth an ace kicker which will redeem most otherwise lousy hands. Where she has neither of these but nonetheless finds herself committed to playing a hand, she will bluff – even to herself.

Male and female interests coincide in that the male wants assurance of paternity whilst the female is defenceless unless he has that assurance and so will play his role. The human female may be insatiable and almost permanently sexually receptive, but indiscriminate availability to every male is an improvident (not to say a tiring) strategy.

It may then be that these peculiar properties of the human female have been the principal driving forces towards structured, mutually dependent social units – polygynous, monogamous, occasionally polyandrous – and so towards civilisation itself.

But wherever we find women freed of such concerns by agnosticism, wealth, contraception and the freedom from censure afforded by a tolerant society, we seem to find them claiming an older and more fundamental birthright and flinging themselves into orgiastic sexual practices without reserve.

The Judaeo-Christian tradition manifests an almost palpable terror of women. Subordination to man and the pains of childbirth were woman's punishment for Eve's sin. Babylonian, Egyptian and

Hebrew fears of 'uncleanness' – probably genuinely related to hygiene in the first instance – were transmuted into rigorous proscriptions by the Christian fathers and the early mediaeval church.

Sex between couples was forbidden not only during daylight hours at any season and on the nights preceding Sundays and holy days, but also on Tuesday and Thursday nights and throughout the three forty-day periods of fasting and abstinence in the liturgical year. All contact was also banned during menstruation and for three months preceding and forty days after childbirth.

If, incredibly, rarity occasionally enhanced male pleasure in sex, it can have done precious little for female, nor, indeed, was pleasure considered desirable. St Jerome maintained that the only purpose of marriage was to breed virgins and so populate heaven, and that of its nature it turned man into a fornicator. If a man enjoyed coupling, he made a prostitute of his wife.

Yet the insatiability of women – acknowledged by the Taoists in their belief in woman as an infinite source of *yin* energy and only recently reasserted by the likes of Mary Jane Sherfey (evolutionary selection has left women still capable of enjoying twenty orgasms in an hour) – was recognised, albeit with terror rather than approval, even then. Woman was carnal, weak and the occasion of sin. It was man's duty to contain her sexuality and to protect her at once from herself and from other men.

She must choose liberty without such protection or protection with confinement. Often the latter, which conferred status as well as security, was preferable.

The only women of substance of whose sexual adventures we ever hear are prostitutes, the exceptional, eccentric women who were rich in their own right or, of course, noblewomen, married but engaged in socially acceptable adultery, usually after the provision of an heir and a spare.

Of course, there were available women aplenty at orgies, but these were mostly prostitutes – or, at least, that is how they were designated by their proper sisters.

In fact, almost every urban woman (the rural tradition was always far more mutually supportive and so free and easy, and appears to have retained the indiscriminate ancestral blow-out at least once a year) who became pregnant out of wedlock, or, as a nurse, domestic servant, seamstress, shop-assistant or whatever, permitted herself to be seduced and yet remained – voluntarily or otherwise – single, was thus designated.

In 1839, Michael Ryan estimated the number of prostitutes in London, a city with a population of two million, at 80,000 – roughly one for every eight sexually active and financially independent males. It is clear that this figure must have included not only every raddled tickle-tail and drab, every champagne-swilling tart at Kate Hamilton's and every high-class 'pretty horsebreaker' who counted dukes and princes amongst her protectors, but also every dollymop – the ambivalent name for every sexually active nurse, nursemaid, servant-girl, *midinette* (which had the same nudge-nudge connotations as 'dollymop'), dancer, artist's model, actress and barmaid.

Many such women were indeed – or soon perforce became – more or less prostitutes. Without a protector (who might as well be a pimp or brothel-madam as an affectionate gentleman or tradesman), incomes for single women were insufficient to sustain life.

The female *demimonde*, then, to which the male *monde* could resort was enormous, but single women who wanted sexual diversity must risk ruin.

The only exceptions to this rule – then as throughout history – were queens, empresses and their immediate courts and, latterly, millionaires' daughters and film stars. Most of these have made full use of their liberty to enjoy varied and sybaritic sex lives. It is only since ordinary women have enjoyed something akin to economic equality and freedom that swinging has taken off as a *bona fide* social network and lifestyle in its own right.

Many other factors already cited – efficient contraception, extended active life, the Internet, the breakdown of the extended (and the failure of the nuclear) family, the universal acceptance of condoms – have contributed to swinging's phenomenal growth and infiltration of mainstream culture. But it is middle-class women's ability and desire to express and to fulfil sexual fantasy, and the resultant or corollary willingness of middle-class men to seek mutuality in their partnerships, which finally broke the locks – and let loose the dreams.

So that carnality, exhibitionism and insatiable sensuality so dreaded by early Christians and Confucians has not been extinguished by millennia of repression (by women no less than men), but has, it seems, been stirring just below the surface, awaiting the moment when it could lash its giant tail and burst out into the sunlight.

The same would seem to apply to the pervasiveness of homosexual activity in such women. Swinging women are not 'gay', nor would they ever consider that they belong in some distinct sexual subcategory. They are 'normal' women – most of them devoted mothers and wives – who just happen to find other women beautiful and desirable. Bisexual activity in swinging is elective and spontaneous, yet it is the majority preference amongst females.

Unless we are to assume that such critical rebels are all by coincidence identically deviant yet slavish followers of fashion, we must conclude that this is a 'natural' preference when once extraneous inhibiting factors are removed.

5

'ONLY SEX'

I DO NOT KNOW WHY SOME people love sex and so find swinging congenial and engrossing whilst others regard us with incomprehension and, although professing to enjoy sex, nonetheless tell us that it is 'only sex' and are baffled by our preoccupation with it. Strange, that the 'only sex' and the 'sacred sex' contingents are so often the same.

I place little credence in the notion that we are divided into the 'highly sexed' and the 'undersexed'. Of course there are hormonal differences, but women who are clearly awash with oestrogen can be every bit as raunchy as those who give every indication of high testosterone levels, and the butch *poilu* is, so far as I am aware, no more gifted with sexual vigour and passion than the slight, smooth and apparently effeminate male.

Psychological distinctions are clearer and appear to be more influential. It was once fashionable to categorise any psychological factor inhibiting sexuality as a 'hang-up', but there have surely been moments in human history when desire beyond that for occasional marital sex must have been anti-social and a damnable nuisance for the person so afflicted.

It is my belief, however – and I fully accept that I may be deluded and others sane, even as I acknowledge, in the teeth of my own experience, that my excitement at fresh, seasonal food and the messages which it conveys may be due to excessive imagination rather than the food's inherent properties – that the 'only sex' brigade are simply doing it all wrong.

I here run the risk of the derision even of the rational and sympathetic as well as the despite of the 'moral majority', but what the hell?

Sex is supra-linguistic or it is pointless. Any attempt to explore or elucidate it in language is therefore poetry or gibberish, depending on your mood or point of view.

I would argue from personal conviction that the 'twin sperm' theory, generally held until the nineteenth century – whereby a female contributes an equal active principle in the process of conception – is, in all save the dreariest, most literal sense, true of all heterosexual sex.

The notion that the male is subject and the female object, or that merely because semen is emitted in visible jolts it is the sole product and the principal medium of sexual congress, has always seemed to me an incomprehensible and incredible nonsense.

Maybe the female product is more aethereal and less physically quantifiable but, ever since I lost my virginity, I have known that, when I kiss a woman, go down on her or fuck her, she is transferring – transmitting – to me the essence of her past, her present and even her ancestors, that I am receiving through my mouth, my nose, my penis a flood of unutterably precious understanding and information. She is communicating with me at a level far beyond that attainable by any other means.

To be 'good in bed' requires, of course, a certain technical proficiency, but above all, it consists in responsiveness. When we kiss – and I can kiss for hours and hours, totally engrossed – I breathe in her longings, her insecurities, her fantasies and her fears. When I sink my muzzle between her legs, I inhale – I ingest – her innermost longings and deepest secrets.

I certainly do not experience this as fancy. For me, it is as physically real as any seminal ejaculation. The Chinese recognised – or fancied her the same thing in the concept of the inexhaustible resource of revivifying *yin* which flows from the female. At first, that flow is mainstream, sweet, slow and slowly swelling. Then, one by one, the upstream sluices open on a hundred tributaries, bringing coolness, freshness and fragrances bright as sunlight from the upland rivulets of memory. And finally, triumphantly – sometimes long before orgasm but its necessary herald – she opens up and the aethereal flow becomes a flood.

And if, amidst so generous a spate of intimate information, I cannot discern what she wants, how best I can communicate in return, what monsters lurk within her and how I can banish them and take her on a carefree spree – well, 'Lord, thy most pointed pleasure take, and stab my spirit broad awake'.

And yet, how many women have turned to me afterwards and panted 'How did you know?'

How did I know? When a master of wine can distinguish the age and precise region of origin of mere fermented grape-juice, confined in a bottle for years?

Here, by contrast, is a living, vibrant, needy creature expressing everything about herself through this effusion, and we are privileged to savour it for hour upon hour.

And if this is the finest, most mutual and most intense form of communication known to humans, it seems perfectly logical that it should be practised between strangers. The alternative, after all, is a deal of nervous posing, pretence and negotiation – otherwise courtship – which asserts the differences between us rather than our oneness. As well prohibit the exhibition of art until the viewer has had an explanatory conversation with the artist, or forbid conversation until semaphore has been essayed for a prescribed time.

6

KISSING AND FUCKING CONSIDERED AS FINE ARTS

I CANNOT HELP BUT WONDER, then, whether the confusion regarding sex is not in part due to mistaken classification.

It is, after all, conceived of as a sinful activity requiring legal certification and religious sanction. It is a sacramental spiritual experience. It is the signature which makes a contract between two people exclusive and binding. It is a selfish pleasure to be enjoyed at every opportunity regardless of consequences, or a selfish pleasure with due regard to consequences.

Maybe, after all, it should be perceived as an art.

Like all arts, it is a sensual means of communication between otherwise estranged humans.

Like all arts, it affords pleasure, joy and enlightenment or, at its best, transcendence and awareness of the essential unity binding otherwise disparate beings.

Like all arts, it requires high craft, self-discipline, sensitivity and passion.

Like all arts, it has its enormously gifted, dedicated and responsive practitioners, compelled to communicate by this means and to perfect their skills, and its everyday, modest practitioners whose amateurish efforts are appreciated only by themselves and their nearest and dearest.

It is thus, like all arts, at once trivial, playful and of the first importance – and surely as valid in an ensemble as in a mere pairing.

And for us who are compulsive, passionate artists – good or bad but never indifferent – the notion of restriction to one audience and one subject is little short of an outrage.

7

THE FREEDOM OF FORGIVENESS

THE PERSISTENT PREREQUISITES OF popular pornography – the 'cumshot', the gleeful bathing in, and consumption of, semen, the bisexual threesomes and moresomes, the lesbian pseudo-coupling – indicate a prevailing theme in visions of sexual pleasure in our culture. It is that of forgiveness.

Those with more prejudice than wit will identify these as glorifying or aggrandising the male role and functions in sex. So, in a sense, they do, but the male starts from an altogether inglorious and ignominious position.

From childhood onward, the female is presented to him (and maybe it is in part an innate perception of the life-giving mother rather than merely convention) as perfect, mysterious, daunting and invariably giving or selling her love to the worthy rather than needing to receive it. Beauty itself is 'immaculate', 'perfect', 'pure'. The intruder is always the criminal or, at best, the inferior guest. As for the guest who 'takes' something from the house and leaves stains on the carpet ...

As his sexuality develops, he must betray this high ideal. His body has long been a polluter and an object of shame, incurring by its wilful emissions embarrassment and increased laundry bills. A girl's body stirs secretly, a boy's overtly. A girl may dirty bed sheets, but she is guiltless. The waxy streaks left by a boy's body, however, betray the yearnings of his unconscious mind no less than of his body.

In adolescence (and, far too often, long afterward), his dreams are a battlefield between those polarised images of Madonna and whore which are so central to our culture, and his loyalties shift from one to the other according to the impulses of his body.

The coexistence of Madonna and whore in one entity (the reality) is an impossibility, a nonsense, as is confirmed at every turn by the iconography of religion, literature and the media and, of course, the image projected by the asexual mother herself. His own sexuality will not permit such a concept. He cannot masturbate or fuck whilst his pitying or disapproving mother looks on.

So, as with Stephen Dedalus in Joyce's *Portrait of the Artist as a Young Man*, the adolescent boy must soar to celestial heights and plummet to infernal depths. When he elects to side with his nascent sexuality, he must become iconoclast and scar and betray the beautiful object of aspiration. When he is 'spiritual', he must renounce and despise the succubi who formerly dragged him down. And it is his shameful, demanding, pollutant genitals which create this conflict.

Pornography, however, resolves it – albeit briefly. The porn star remains iconic, intangible, ideal and unmarred by his lusts because on a screen or a page. Christ-like, however, she descends from the aethereal regions to become incarnate, to sanction, to share and even to love man's destructive urges. She feasts upon his pollutant organs and ejaculate. She emulates him with other women. She smiles gleefully and joins in, complicit, as other males fuck other women. A celestial combination of *noli me tangere* and *et vir facta est*.

And so the supposedly irreconcilable poles of woman and man, purity and sexuality, ideal and gross, find a bridge in pornography. It is the ultimate Manichean genre.

Many women deem pornography exploitative and, indeed, blame the men whom they perceive as its principal consumers (they would prefer that they were its only consumers) for abusing women. Of course, in certain specific cases, this is true. In general, however, it is those women who depend upon the robes, regalia and decorum of a mythical power who now resent their sisters who have renounced them.

The porn star, like the swinger, does not set aside the robes of state to affect undignified grungy male clothes or stained and squalid tatters. She steps forward naked, crying, as it were, *'hypocrite voyeur, mon semblable, mon frère!'*, and is no less magnificent, nurturing or mighty than those who elect to hide their humanity, just as the human Jesus is no less venerable than his distant and daunting Father. She retains, however, an alternate intangibility – a glamour – by means of the effects of cinema or video.

Porn affords the illusion of forgiveness for what has for so long been condemned, not least by the archetypes of the female gender, and forgiveness is the ultimate liberation for one reared and educated in self-despite and self-disgust.

But then, that is precisely what female swingers also tell me about their experience of swinging. Again and again, they report enormous relief, the lifting of a burden, a sense of acceptance and validation of aspects of their bodies and their souls which they have felt obliged to keep concealed for decades. They too are at last forgiven for being whole and female.

If both genders then seek pardon for being what they unavoidably are, perhaps we should concede that religion is right in considering our bodily functions dirty and reprehensible. Or perhaps – just perhaps – we should consider that it is the guilt and shame which are sick and wrong, that the transitory sense of liberation afforded by pornography is therapeutic, and that afforded by socially ordered swinging positively healthy.

Swinging renders pornography redundant for both genders. Here sex and sexual fantasy are shared, celebrated and adored as glorious, vital, playful and pleasurable aspects of human being.

I confess that this is, for me, the principal joy of swinging.

To sit at a computer console with a girl, plotting sexual adventures and selecting playmates or parties, to plan her outfit for a night out, to hold hands and kiss, or wink at one another as we play with others, to discuss our experiences afterwards, to laugh together over them and to fuck stimulated by pride and the awareness of one another as alive, fallible, powerful, beautiful and yes, *semblable* – even *frère* and *soeur* – this is a sort of free, easy, unabashed companionship denied to others who are separated, rather than united, by their genders and their fantasies.

I look forward to my next close and, with luck, enduring relation-ship with as much wistfulness and enthusiasm as any teenage girl dreaming of 'the love of her life', but I find it hard now to conceive of such a relationship without the equality, companionship and openness which I have known through swinging partnerships.

PART IX

1

ALL THAT GLISTERS ...

I HAD AT FIRST THOUGHT TO COMPILE a precise, restaurant-style guide to the regular clubs and parties which my partners and I have visited here and abroad.

Not only did I realise, however, that this must soon be unjust and inaccurate – clubs and parties come and go, change management and improve or worsen – but, although I generally disdain relativism, preferences here are peculiar and peculiarly personal. Far more than in gastronomy, in which we can at least declare ingredients and preparation to be good or bad, sexuality admits of an almost infinite number of individual predilections.

Catt, for example, an otherwise refined 36-year-old blonde who has often stayed with us with her eager, voyeuristic, non-participant husband, asks us to organise quasi-rape scenarios in public places for her – six men and Katy in a graffiti-daubed subway (our driving-instructor friend Alan enjoyed surprising her. He was the drooling, genuinely stinking tramp crouched close by who at last joined in the fun), a similar scene in the dunes at Braunton, another in an Exeter multi-storey car-park. Hardly standard notions of luxurious pleasure.

So too, our friends Donna and Dave favour a club called the Office in Bristol. I hate it.

Located on the unused second floor of an office block in an insalu-brious area, the Office's décor reminds me of a provincial university's junior common room whose entertainments officer has been entrusted with £200 to deck it out for an 'erotica'-themed evening. Inflatable penises, fishnets (the actual nets rather than hose), formica-topped tables and a sticky revolving bed which has not revolved within living memory are amongst the results.

The place is popular with unconvincing transvestites. The single males who haunt it seem to me peculiarly unattractive and have a poorly developed sense of body-distance. They play with themselves with far more enthusiasm than themselves would seem to warrant ...

But then, I am a sensualist and a snob (strange, that I still shudder from excessive proximity to the clothed multitude on a tube train, yet will happily play naked amidst hundreds of strangers), whereas Donna freely admits that this rough and ready, basement bar ethos is part of the turn-on for her.

No party, too, is ever quite the same from one occasion to another. We have returned to the same location as that at which we previ-ously enjoyed a wonderful, oblivious orgy and an entertaining social evening, only to find that guests are tethered in the kitchen, the con-versation is hesitant and nervous and only a few of us dare shed clothes.

Equally, we have attended parties where, at first sight, the guests put me in mind rather of the darkest recesses of rock-pools than of my sexual fantasies, yet where we have found one or two couples or singles who have made the evening memorable and worthwhile.

Even at the Office, Sally and I once found the most delightful, sensuous, amusing and loving couple – alas, soft swingers who have yet to relent – and spent hours blissfully enravelled with them. They have since become good friends. They have not induced us to return to their home club.

2

BIRMINGHAM – A MODEL

DIFFERENT CLUBS AND PARTIES have different purposes and appeal to different people. There are three swingers' clubs in or near Birmingham which conveniently illustrate some of the alternatives. They are all excellent, but they all serve different purposes.

Many swingers love Xtasia in West Bromwich. The place is well-run, spotlessly clean and ideal for socialising swingers wishing to meet others. Essentially, however, this is a nightclub with added-on facilities for play. The focus is the disco dance floor, noisy and cramped as all such dance floors are. Every half hour, the music slows, a curtain falls about the dancers, single males must step out and a general grope-fest ensues.

It is all very jolly. I have played in the spa area and in the lounge. In the basement, too, there is a police box or 'tardis' whose walls are pierced with 'glory-holes', where once (perhaps because most of me was invisible) I had hours' worth of lavish attention from a succession of women (Sally was charged with ensuring that they *were* women and attractive, since I could see nothing save lips and arses throughout).

But I am a sybarite and an experienced orgiast. I prefer to get lost in my lovers and in the moment. I love the freedom of the orgy, in which newcomers can be welcomed into the party and one's arms, and players can sprawl, relax and chat between bouts of vigorous activity.

Every area and alcove at Xtasia seems to have different rules or conditions of entry. You have to dress and undress again and again. The play areas are cramped and sometimes uncomfortable.

It is, however, a first-rate club for those wanting confidence, seeking to meet new friends or simply to observe swingers, and a comfortable, very swinger-friendly hotel nearby is where the serious play starts afterwards.

Utopia near Telford has just about everything that a swinging couple could desire. It is housed in a mansion, with all the advantages and disadvantages which that presupposes. The advantages include the grandeur and sense of luxury of the venue which are worthy of any top-class hotel or country-club – a fifteen-metre indoor pool overlooked by an eight-person jacuzzi, a steam room, plenty of private rooms, two very comfortable lounges, a couples' playroom and a dark room. It is easy to avoid any scene or group that does not appeal.

The problem is that you can easily lose the party in all that space. A network of greenish fibreglass caves was installed in Utopia's earlier incarnation as a gay club. Each of these can accommodate two friendly couples. If the private rooms are filled and the steam room and swimming pool are busy, a visitor standing in the bar may wonder just where the party has gone whilst two or three hundred people are in fact disporting close at hand. There is also a hardcore clique of regulars which tends to gather in the lounges and makes little effort to engage new friends.

That said, this is a great club for novices, and many people are not here to play save with one another and to watch us less inhibited players. Where else, after all, can you enjoy such facilities with BYOB drink, good company and live, unscripted porn all about you for just £35 per couple per night? This makes it a justifiably popular night out for mainstream vanillas.

We have tended to gravitate to the principal downstairs playroom and the corridor room outside, where play is often varied and abundant. The staff can be really quite outstandingly friendly. If all box-office staff were as generous and playful as Dawn (alas, under previous management), all auditoria would be empty ...

Chameleons, as I have already said, is my favourite British club. If Utopia recalls a country house hotel, 'Chams' is an antiquarian book shop of a sex-club, with lots of different themed rooms on its three levels. The party is at all times all around you. You can wander along the corridors and pick the group which you want to join or the theme which meets your mood.

Although many of the women remain in underwear or skimpy sarongs – and stockings and stilettos, of course – all the men and many of the other women strip on arrival, place their clothes in secure lockers and wear nothing but towels (if that) throughout the remainder of the visit. Like the Polynesian *pareu*, the towel may be worn by women around the waist or around the breasts.

This undress makes the atmosphere relaxed and precludes the often daunting moment when a couple must dare to strip or must fumble around for knickers and socks after playing. Lynne, the manageress, is neither intrusive nor obtrusive, but keeps a weather-eye on everything in her labyrinthine club.

Downstairs, there is a spacious, fully licensed bar and social area and, at the back, a giant jacuzzi in a grotto. On the first floor, there is a lounge – the only one at a swing-club which boasts comfortable seating, pot plants, coffee tables, etc and a television but, blessedly, no porn, so that you can actually catch up with the cricket or watch *Singin' in the Rain* mid-orgy – the red playroom, in which we have spent many wonderful hours, various private rooms and the steam room.

Upstairs again there is the cage-room, where couples play on cushions within an elevated cage or in the best sex-swing in the world, the mirrored couples-room which has a glassed-off viewing area for the voyeurs (this too is often filled with writhing, panting couples inspired by the view), the sauna and, along a narrow dark corridor, the dungeon, which is decidedly unmenacing and boasts another, inferior swing.

Our every Saturday night at Chams has been a long glorious, play-filled night with many partners, but we have always felt impelled, on arising late on the Sunday, to return for further play before heading home. The few single males here know that they are privileged and behave accordingly. Unless specifically invited over by a female or couple, they give players a discreet berth.

There are some prerequisites, then, for a good swing-club or party – cleanliness, cordiality, attentive hosts and social and sexual stimuli close at hand rather than too disparately spread are just four of these – but, even given these, the success or otherwise of a party lies in the hands of the guests.

At present, then, of English clubs, I would unhesitatingly recommend AbFab near Heathrow, La Chambre in Sheffield, Swingers' Junction at Totton near Southampton, Skinny Dippers in Brighton, the Townhouse near Tranmere on the Wirral, the Toucan Club and Coupleszone in London and Fever and Fervour Parties in London and Manchester, but each is as good as its partygoers on the night, each may change, and there are plenty of others which I have not had the chance to explore.

3

FUN4TWO

THE CONTINENTAL EUROPEANS do theatrical erotic luxury better than the British and the North Americans. One day, I may write of the revealing cultural differences manifest in swinging practices worldwide. For now, I must restrict myself – and that all too briefly – to the European swingers' mecca, Fun4Two near Rotterdam.

This is unquestionably the glitziest, most glamorous public club in Europe (I specify 'public' because the most conspicuous celebrities have their own, rather more secretive scene), and is frequented by more than its fair share of beautiful, confident and attractive swingers. The owners have decked the club out in much the same free, frivolous and fanciful way in which swinging women dress for parties. There is no rococo reserve here, nor should there be. It is a nigh universal fantasy of sensual pleasure laid upon sensual pleasure.

There are seventeen different erotically themed rooms here, including a miniature replica of Amsterdam's red light district, a 'sex theatre', an orgy loft and a gloriously lavish 'Tantra Temple' with beautiful and highly skilled masseurs and maseuses to sooth and stimulate players between their exertions.

There is also an outdoor swimming pool, an inside whirlpool jacuzzi, a rather wonderful steam bath and a dance floor. The buffet in the restaurant is, unlike that generally on offer at swing-clubs, genuinely superb. Visits to Fun4Two should be regarded like visits to Disneyland, where fantasies (rather more pleasurably than at Disneyland) become – well, slightly more tangible fantasies. It is far too reliably good to be sustained.

Nights at Fun4Two have invariably been memorably exciting, but in truth, lavish conditions – though fun – are no more guarantees of great experience than more workaday conditions indicate inevitable disappointment.

One late July night, Katy and I discovered heaven right here in Somerset – not merely swingers' heaven, but the compensatory paradise promised to millions of warriors, celibates and dutiful spouses throughout history and dreamed of by every halfway human male adolescent, South Seas traveller, pornography-watcher and artist worthy of the name.

Here were lavish sexual licence and luxury without consequence. Here were visual and sensory delights in abundance. Here were warmth, friendliness and beauty.

And, having found paradise, we rejected it, and found ourselves longing for earth.

4

PARADISE REJECTED

THE ADVERTISEMENT ON Hedonism.co.uk had long intrigued us. It sounded fantastic. We duly disbelieved its claims.

'We are Greg (36, 5'11", athletic) and Natalia (26, 6'1", long-legged, Russian, totally gorgeous, very bi),' it announced. And there indeed was a full-colour picture of a woman with long dark brown or black hair and a dazzling smile. She was slender as a greyhound, and her naked legs, which straddled another slim, beautiful girl in an expensive House of Harlot corset and fishnets, were worthy of any chorusline.

They had built, it seemed, a fantasy tree-house overlooking the lake in their garden and specifically designed for orgies. Their party was by invitation only. There was no charge for admission

It was plain that this – a party held monthly near Priddy – was an exclusive event. None of the swingers whom we had met at other parties had ever attended it. Few knew of its existence. Greg and Natalia, it seemed, must invite London and international friends to their rural retreat.

I do not know whether it was our cosmopolitanism, Katy's youth or my academic background which won us an invitation. We received a request for pictures and, shortly afterwards, a call on my mobile from an urbane, well-spoken Englishman who called himself 'Tony'. He twanged Leslie Phillips or James Hewitt style, just a little bit too much to be a gentleman, but it was close. Although he said that he was merely a friend of the family, Tony invited us to the party the following Saturday and asked us to come 'specially early so that we could look around.

We arrived that evening at a very isolated country house. It was long, low and white, a once modest little farmhouse which had spawned, for it now had a family clustered around it – a single-storey extension which clung to its apron strings at its right, a burly double garage at its left, a flighty little thatched gazebo on the opposite bank and, up to the house's right, half-hidden amongst maples, a log cabin with a veranda all about it and long stilts which reached down to a lake crowded with shrubs.

As we climbed out of the car and looked about us, we could see nothing of the rural setting. We might have been in a very grand sub-urban garden. It was plain, too, that this was a garden so laboriously created and jealously tended that no part of it was to be stolen on vis-itors' shoes. Decking walkways snaked from the sub-tropical section to the water-garden, from the water-garden to the rockery, from the rockery to the arboretum.

Some people look tall, others short, regardless of height. The bald, sketch-bearded man who emerged from the front door, his right hand extended and already clasping something invisible, was of the short variety. His wife did not help. She followed close behind him, and, although only a couple of inches taller, seemed to tower over him. She wore a skin-tight black garment which, to quote Tom Wolfe, 'fingered into every fissure' and patent shoes with stilettos which would skewer a Schwarzenegger's heart. Her body was lean, limber, long-legged – beautiful.

She was really, it seemed, called Tanya. Her hair was black and glossy. Her smile was broad. Her face was classically pretty. She leaned forward to kiss us, first one by one on the lips, then, pulling our heads together, both of us simultaneously. I glimpsed the foundation which refused to crease at quite the same rate as the lines on her forehead, the lines between the wings of her sweet little nose and the corners of her mouth. She looked stunning, but hers was a coked-up showgirl's beauty. For 26, at close quarters and in daylight, she looked bloody awful.

'So good you come!' she enthused. 'So good!' Her hands trailed along our forearms as she stepped backward.

Greg spoke in a flattened South London accent. 'Yeah. Great you guys could make it.'

They gave us the guided tour of the garden. 'And we put the lake in ...' Greg said airily. 'We've only been 'ere eight years ... wasteland when we found it.

'We just built this place like we'd always wanted a playroom to be,' he said as we neared the log cabin. 'The routine is, around 10, all the girls change into lawnjeray. The music gets pretty loud, so, if you go outside for any reason, don't leave the door open, OK? Nearest neighbour's three miles away, but we still get complaints ...'

He held open the door. I caught Katy's eye. We both hate repetitive music which hijacks your pulse and natural rhythms. A moment later, we had forgotten all such qualms. We were turning about, scanning the room, behaving for all the world like first-time tourists in the Pantheon.

The wall at our right had been faced with rough grey stone. It accommodated a stone fireplace in which a spitted ox would fit with ease. Above the fireplace, there hung a huge painting of our host, apparently in a gilt throne in this very room, with naked girls kneeling or sitting at his feet.

The wall opposite us was plate glass, overlooking the lake and the gazebo on the opposite bank. The window-seat was deeply upholstered. Huge cushions fringed with gold lay propped along its length.

At our left, taking up a good third of the room's floor space, was the biggest bed that I have ever seen – a six-poster, four times king-sized, with a wall of dark, mottled mirror behind its putative head. Flickering torches leaned from sconces on each carved post. More torches burned along the walls. At either end of the bed, there was a dancing pole on a small circular platform.

'You'll find boxes under there for your things,' said Greg, 'Just make one yours when you get undressed ... Now, I've got to get this fire lit. Tan, babes, you take them down to the house and get them a drink, OK?'

Tanya put her arms around our waists and allowed us to lead her back to the house. She showed us into a huge, crypt-like, arched kitchen.

The couples standing about, to whom we were introduced as we entered, were all fit, well-groomed and beautiful. There was Renata, a tall blonde Estonian woman of perhaps 30 in a little black dress, and her man Marius, dark, athletic, tanned and perhaps five years her senior. There was Elena in short, silky green, maybe 26, again with a slender dancer's body, hair the colour of Indian tea and lovely, prob-ing, pale grey eyes. Her man, Jason, was of the wire and whipcord variety, with a sharp, eager, drawn but attractive face.

Then, sitting at the table, there were two girls, Pavla and Marie-Louise – one from Slovakia, the other from London. Pavla had raven's wing hair, swooping raven eyebrows and a broad, laughing mouth. She wore a tight, lacy scarlet top and a scarlet frou-frou skirt. Marie-Louise – the only English girl there – had long, honey-coloured hair and at present, wore nothing beyond a shimmery little grey negligee and – her right foot was on the chair beside her left thigh, her chin laid on her raised knee, so we were left in no doubt – grey satin cami-knickers trimmed with white lace.

These figures were distracting and surprising enough – figures from a swingers' theme park or a very, very superior porn movie. The man at the head of the table belonged obviously in neither. He might have come from a seventies' thriller, though. He too was slim, glossy and well turned-out, with perfectly trimmed, swept-back hair, a double-cuffed, blue striped poplin shirt with oval gold links, and well-manicured hands. The signet on his little finger was well worn. The glittering Rolex spoke louder, and of newer money.

'Tony Van Santen,' he drawled, standing as we entered. He then sat and leaned back, crossing fawn-clad legs. His socks were long and sheer. 'Sit down, sit down. Delighted you could make it.' He made the various introductions. This was the 'family friend', but he behaved as though he owned the place and everyone in it.

He was gracious and charming. I guessed, given his age, which I put at mid-forties, that he had ridden the Thatcherite bore in the early eighties. There was a trace of cruelty in those thin lips, a glint of steel in those pale, amber-haloed grey eyes. He was a lawyer, he said, though he was obviously too glossy ever to have practised as a solicitor and too obviously furtive even for the bar. He owned a company which financed and developed new medical apparatus. He also owned, as we concluded later, a whole lot more.

There were now ten women and nine men aside from us and our hosts. All the girls were confident, warm, gentle and welcoming in manner. All had beautiful legs. Eight of them were from Central or Eastern Europe. The men were rougher in manner, but all were polite, muscular and apparently fit, and all plainly had money to burn.

Perhaps we should have cottoned on before Tony told us that it was time to change and to make our way up to the playhouse. We were just too delighted to find ourselves in such company and in such a location. Who now wanted Secrets with its often middle-aged women and their often shrunken husbands? I had made definite eye-contact with four of the girls. Katy was playing underwear-inspection girly games with the women and positively squirming at the men.

Up there in that beautiful room, the music was pounding and the mist from the smoke machine rising. We danced and embraced and caressed one another. Even then, we did not notice that the dancing was just too good, that the girls on the poles were entwining themselves about them too smoothly and sinuously, doing the splits like ballerinas and hanging head down with the ease of fruit bats.

We did notice that they snorted a lot of coke off the marble-topped console tables at either side of the fireplace, that they kept changing outfits, and that each new corset, teddy or bra and panties set was gorgeous and fitted perfectly, but that all fitted in with the sense that we were playing in a pornographic ballet and were no longer of the real, dreary world.

We fell onto that big bed and started to play. Tanya and Elena joined us there. They kissed us, licked us, sucked us. Their bodies were beautiful. They were both great kissers. They were both genuinely bisexual. There was a lot of kissing, caressing and, almost incidentally, fucking in there.

Tony, now naked, knelt behind Elena and fucked her as she played with Katy. He wasn't wearing a condom. I was mildly surprised, but assumed, in so far as I was capable of reasoning by now, that she was a peculiarly close and trusted friend. He pulled out of her ... Tanya turned away from me to suck his cock, then presented her upraised rump to him. Again he entered her too without a condom.

By now, other couples were playing around us. I took stock. There was Katy being fucked by Marius whilst eating Renata. I moved towards them. Katy raised her head and kissed me with a tongue and lips by now deliciously and diversely sauced. Renata joined us in the kiss and went down on me ... and so on ...

For a while there it seemed as though we were about to fly off into that timeless orgiastic ecstasy, that blissful defiance of the gravity of individual identity, propriety and responsibility which marks true play. But something was tethering me to earth. I was self-conscious and wary. I felt that we were intruders, that we were watched. I felt an obscure sense of menace.

Marie-Louise, the blonde London girl, joined us. We kissed and began to fuck, very gently. Her body spoke of aching need. Beside us, Tony knelt between Katy's legs. She raised her knees. He shuffled between them and thrust his hips forward. She slapped a hand over her labia and mouthed, 'Condom!'

He tutted. The corner of his lips twitched. He glanced over his shoulders as if looking for a dilatory condom-bearing steward. He sighed and glared almost disdainfully down at Katy, then turned away. Katy crawled over to lie at Marie-Louise's side until we separated.

She said, 'Hey, take a break?' Her eyes were full of alarm.

I nodded. I kissed Marie-Louise. I said, 'Right, we're going to get a breath of fresh air.'

'Are you OK?' Marie-Louise wanted to know. She grasped our hands and looked up at us.

'Sure,' I smiled. 'Just a bit ...'

'Just a bit hot in here,' supplied Katy. She too bent to kiss the naked girl.

The two of us gathered our underwear from the boxes under the bed. By now, the bed resembled a pond during frog-mating season, so our departure would pass, I assumed, unnoticed. I followed Katy out onto the walkway. We shut the noise in and breathed in the relative silence. Still carrying our underclothes, we walked down a flight of wooden stairs to a lower level where we perched above the lake. Katy sat at my right and leaned against me. I hugged her. I kissed the top of her head.

'I want to leave,' she said.

'So do I,' I admitted. 'It's so bloody unfair!'

'I know. It's fucking perfect, but something's wrong ...'

'What is it?'

'I don't know. I think they're all owned by Tony. I mean, where's Greg in all this? What is he? Some type of muscle employed by Tony? These girls – I mean, they're sweet, but could they argue if they wanted to? They're like pros ...'

'And this place ...' I waved at the garden, the throbbing playhouse above us. 'It's all wrong ...'

There was a clatter behind us. Marie-Louise had followed us. Naked but for stockings and high heels, she sauntered across the walkway, squatted down, put an arm around my neck and reached her other hand out to Katy. I felt her lips on the nape of my neck and her breasts soft and warm on my back.

'You guys feeling a bit intimidated?' she asked.

'I suppose,' I shrugged.

'Freaked out more like,' said Katy. 'I mean, you're all lovely, this place is lovely, but what's the story? Whose is this place? Where have you all sprung from? What's with Tony and no condoms?'

'No point in asking me!' she laughed. 'I just come along and enjoy the fun. Makes a nice break. I mean, Greg owns the place, but I think all the extensions, the playhouse, all this – I think all that was Tony's doing. They diverted the river, you know, extended the gardens, built all this, all without planning permission ... Cost a quarter of a million ...'

'And they know full well that it would take just one complaint by an aggrieved neighbour and they'd lose the lot ...' I mused. 'So a lot of cash they don't mind losing because it's not real money. There's nowhere else for it to go ...'

'Maybe. I just don't ask questions.' Marie-Louise sat at my left side. She too rested a head on my shoulder. 'It's lovely, though, isn't it?'

'Oh, it's great ...'

'You're pretty good on that pole,' said Katy dreamily.

'Years of practice. I used to be at Spearmint Rhinos. Still do a few nights a month, and train the girls ...'

'Girls?'

'Yep. Bernie's got three London clubs.'

'Are you all – are most of you ex-dancers?'

She sighed. 'Yep, I think so. We're the lucky ones. Married the bosses.'

'What about Tanya?' I asked.

'Oh, poor Tans. No. Don't know where Greg found her. Model, I think. He keeps her down here all week, poor thing. Staff to do everything. She lives for these weekends. Gets to see us, have a bit of fun at last ...'

'Yes, but Tony,' Katy frowned. 'Where does he fit in?'

'Oh, I don't know, babes! I'd sooner not ask. Just he says "Jump", everyone jumps. He's the lawyer, backer, fixer, lays on these things ...'

She was sweet. Katy and I made her promise to call us. She promised. She came back with us to the playroom and explained to Tony, as we collected the rest of our clothes, that a mythical babysitter had left a message about an imaginary daughter on the house phone. The mobile did not work in the valley, so we had to return to the house to await a return call.

We were back in the kitchen, collecting our coats. Greg was in there, still dressed and busying himself with drinks and rinsing out glasses. Another couple with whom we had not played sat dishevelled at the table, cutting and snorting lines.

Tanya lurched in, singing happily, looking unutterably beautiful and totally mad. She now wore nothing but a little blue-grey silk dressing-gown with a hot pink lining. The belt was untied. 'Hello, everyone!' she said. She slumped down into a chair. 'Hi, Greg. More!'

Greg faintly smiled. He pulled a half-empty Vittel bottle from the fridge, raised a shot glass to the light and squinted as he poured out a good jolt of clear liquid. He delivered the glass to Tanya. She said 'Mmm,' threw back her head and waved her magnificent black mane from side to side. Her smile was still happy and girlish. She drank. Her tongue slowly licked her lips. She shuddered and giggled. 'So good! You want some?'

'What is it?'

'GHB,' she said. 'Is yummy!'

I shook my head. My generation did coke, but I dredged my memory and recalled GHB – gamma hydroxy butyrate – paint-stripper mixed with drain-cleaner which serves as a euphoric, disin-hibiting date-rape drug, 'liquid ecstasy', usually taken in bottle caps, not knocked back like vodka.

'But you have clothes!' Tanya objected. She pouted at me. She opened her legs, licked her middle finger and slid it between her shaven labia. 'I want sex,' she announced. 'You fuck me again?'

I smiled politely. I turned to Katy. She shrugged faintly and nodded. Greg said, 'Go on, mate. She needs it ...' The girl sitting next to me grabbed my cock and said, 'Yes. Come on. I'll help. Poor Tan. Are you a gentleman or not?'

She was right. Noblesse obliged. I knelt and licked that pretty, pouting, flavourless pussy. The other girl knelt behind me, lowered my trousers and caressed my cock and balls. Katy wandered over and kindly laid a hand on the nape of my neck. Greg and the other man discussed local roads.

Eventually, Tanya keened 'Ai' again and again on a rising scale and her groin bucked and slithered all over my face.

I knelt up, raised those long, long legs and fucked her. Her arms wrapped around me, pulling me tight to her. She said, 'Yes, baby. Yes! Harder!' The girl behind me crooned, 'That's it, baby. Good boy! Go on! Fuck her! Harder!' Greg asked, 'Is that good, hun? He good?' then returned to talk of traffic bottlenecks in Farrington Gurney. Katy breathed, 'We've got to go, you know ...'

It was all very surreal and pornographic – the beautiful, warm body wrapped around me and pressed against me, the hot pussy pulsing about me, the quarry tiles hard and ridged beneath my knees, the people all around, absently urging me on.

I grasped Tanya's hair and pulled her head back hard ... I looked into her grey green eyes. I think I had some idea of compelling her back into awareness, of conveying my own humanity, vulnerability and desperation and recognition of hers. I think I sneered. I think – Oh, all right, I fancied – that there was a moment in which the child in her looked out at me with a need profounder and more enduring than the sexual craving which caused her hips to bob and pestle on me.

Then her eyes glittered. She grit her teeth. Her upper lip curled in a snarl. She opened her mouth wide in a silent laugh. I spat and slammed my hips against her.

Tenderness and worship may tentatively foster union, but the damned are united too, and they get there faster.

Katy said, 'Right, come on, love. We've really got to get moving.'

In the back of the taxi on the way back, she cuddled up in my arms and shuddered. 'God, that was weird.'

'Yep.' I kissed her. 'Really sad. All those girls owned by their husbands.'

'All those men owned by that sleazebag, Tony. I mean, I think the girls all actually enjoyed it. Ex-dancers, some of them probably high-class working-girls, now confined to quarters as trophy wives for gangsters or whatever ... Must be a break for them. God, they could have drugged us, raped us, disappeared us if they'd wanted to ...'

'Nasty. Very nasty.' I hugged her to me as she shuddered again. 'And you were the one who said all those ordinary people with ordinary bodies at Secrets were a turn-off ...'

'I know, and tonight should have been heaven, but I would have killed to be back at Secrets with real people just having fun.'

She shook her head against me as though to worry a hole in my chest. Then she waxed philosophical. Her question echoed a thousand folk and fairy tales. 'Oh, why does heaven on earth always seem to be really hell?'

5

HAVING YOUR CAKE AND
EATING IT

SO NEITHER GILT, PLUSH nor lissom, lovely bodies are guarantees of successful orgies, nor, alas, good animate eating of worthy inanimate foodstuffs. In fact, the usual fare at good parties and bad alike is of the pre-cooked chicken satay and mini-sausage-roll variety.

So too, some reading this book selectively may think that the very presence of large numbers of raunchy, sensuous, sexually liberated people will automatically mean unbridled indulgence of their own wilder fantasies on their own terms.

So it may, but again I must warn that swinging is not for everyone, not least because it will never be entirely on their own terms. If they cannot attune themselves to others' feelings and fantasies and take pleasure from their fulfilment, they should stick to their favourite porn movies.

They must also abandon certain of the commonplace consolations of middle-class life and assumed identity. For women, swinging entails a willing renunciation of the power afforded by the illusion of virtue and inaccessibility – the identical power to that claimed by the anally retentive child on the pot.

This is brave but realistic. It is from the archetype of 'the Great Mother' – the unblemished, life-giving but awful idol – that modern women have for so long derived their power. Satin evening gowns, cosmetics and soft lighting pretend to the inviolability and smooth homogeneity of the statue. Cracks and fissures need be shown only to a trusted (because presumed captive) few.

Female swingers do not renounce the glamour of glacial composure and surface elegance. Not for them the grungy, sprawling self-despite of Jacobin feminists. They are properly vain, they must have faith rather in the beauty of their functioning, desirous and desirable bodies and in the holiness of their mortal lusts.

'My biggest kick is going back to work on a Monday morning in a business suit, looking cool and in control,' says Christy. 'And all the girls there are talking about whether or not they're going to sleep with this guy or that and whether so-and-so was good in bed or, more usually has lost interest in sex, and I'm just this serene, sympathetic, detached person. If they think about it at all, they probably think I'm celibate.

'But just occasionally, I cross my legs and squeeze and think, "Oh, if only you knew what I was up to on Saturday! All those men, all those girls, all that fun ..." But that's another life. They'll never know. It's mine. And next week, we'll be back there again, and I get all excited, but all they can see is this respectable woman ...'

For men, it requires a willingness to expose themselves and their shortcomings – literal and figurative, imagined and actual – and a readiness to submit to feminine requirements for sensuality and eroticism rather than seeking their own short-term physical gratification.

The man for whom sexual pleasure exists only in the genital area or who considers orgasm its purpose will derive little pleasure from, and will make few friends in, swinging.

For those who are not so handicapped, however, and are willing to be appraised and accepted without props or uniforms and take joy in casting them off, swinging is enormous, adventurous, sociable fun. It is also one of the few remaining shared hobbies accessible to married couples, with all the joys of hunting, anticipation, games-playing and intimacy built in.

For myself, I had too often allowed sexual desire and the longing for company to lead me into relationships which I would not normally have undertaken, with people with whom, in truth, I had little in common save loneliness and a desire for affection and sex.

My partners were usually seeking very different things from our encounters, and the results were unsatisfactory if not obviously injurious.

We were battling to reconcile sexual licence, which was plainly logical and morally unexceptionable, with the assay criteria for self-esteem with which we had been reared.

Those 'assay criteria', many sexologists and historians would argue, were set by frightened males and imposed by religion, social and economic pressures and literary and cinematic convention.

Although the whore/Madonna, dross/sterling dichotomy has been the insulting curse of generations of women, women themselves have found it hard to abandon this absurd bipolarity.

There have been many casualties. In the seventies and eighties, I met many girls who, having sought to respond to the culture's urgings to assert their liberated status and to assuage loneliness by transitory sexual relationships, found themselves therefore downgraded in their immediate societies and – still more seriously – in their own estimation.

On the 'as well be hanged for a sheep as a lamb' principle, they plunged into a maelstrom of self-despite, further transitory reassurance and rebelliousness and further self-despite as the perceived distance between themselves and their early nineteenth-century models grew. Some killed themselves. Some became drunkards or drug addicts. Some merely became sad and bitter.

Men found it easier to reconcile the archetypes of philanderer and 'the marrying kind', because the nineteenth-century model postulated these as the two stages in a man's sexually active life, but these stages were implausibly deemed to be distinct and mutually exclusive. For a woman, no such harmonious 'two-in-one' sequential model existed. She must be saved or damned.

Contemporary men and women are still striving to reconcile these distinct and conflicting aspects of their natures and their conditioning (though 'that was during my wild period' or, 'I went through a self-destructive patch' are now standard phrases in almost every woman's armoury). Some resort to casual sex with all its resultant confusions. Some, like thousands of gays in the past century, marry, try to ignore their ever more exigent impulses and yearnings and almost inevitably fail.

At the last, swinging's critics generally resort to a curious premiss of justice derived rather from Granny's *Olde Booke of Sage Precepts* than from any moral code related to pragmatism or reason. 'Yes, but that can't be right. You're trying to have your cake and eat it.' To which the most telling reply would seem to be, 'Yes? And ...?'

Swingers believe – and, I think, demonstrate – that they can indeed have their cake and eat it, that they can maintain loving, exclusive relationships, self-respect and the respect of their communities whilst enjoying active, varied and adventurous sex lives.

'I just no longer wanted to cause hurt, or to be subject to it,' says Marcus. 'I was sick and tired of the mess and the emotional confusion resulting from exclusive "romance". The Lifestyle seemed clean by comparison: compassionate, companionable, amusing and affectionate.

'For all the occasional crassness and vulgarity of some of those involved, for all the occasional moments when – not generally because of the nature of swinging but because of my own state of mind – the whole business has seemed a bit squalid and silly, I've never had cause to change my mind about that.'

6

'THAT FRIVOLOUS PRETENCE ...'

'Tell me no more of constancy.
That frivolous pretence,
Of cold age, narrow jealousy,
Disease and want of sense ...'[2]

ROCHESTER'S DISDAINFUL APPRAISAL of sexual continence as a symptom of debility or cowardice rings out across the centuries, magnificent and defiant as that of any rebel against a smug and craven establishment.

In an age of incurable pox and unreliable contraception, it may actually have been rather less splendid. Today, however, with sexually transmitted disease readily contained or cured and conception preventable, his views are worthy of consideration.

---

[2]John Wilmot, Earl of Rochester, 'Tell Me No More of Constancy', *The Poems*, ed. K Walker, Oxford: Oxford University Press, 1984

Sexual desire is, after all, an appetite, its means of gratification as diverse as the partners with whom it can be attained and shared. I am not talking about orgasm, which is a physiological function and – although variable in intensity – tends always to be essentially the same, but of the endless sensory pleasures – the sights, sounds, scents, tastes and sensations which presage, accompany, enhance and often transcend the so-called 'sexual act' between two or more people.

So food, once in the belly – though its long-term effects may differ – is just undifferentiated substance. The glutton seeks only the faintly repugnant sensations of repletion. To the gastronome, however, each individual item of food – each fruit, flower, vegetable, fish and cut of meat – is unique. Combine each with others, have due regard to context and provenance, relish the anticipation, the fragrances, the visual properties, the conflicting, contrasting and harmonious textures and savours of each, and we have one of the supremely civilised joys of human existence.

So although we may with very good reason despise the glutton, who merely seeks to stuff his or her belly, who would reprove the passionate chef or gourmet who spends life in heightened awareness of the possibilities afforded by God's lavish and profuse creation, and infinite curiosity as to its uses?

When the same question is asked of sexual connoisseurship, responses are very odd. Those for whom such exploration is – for reasons temperamental, moral or physical – repugnant, seem to find some consolation in the assertion that the 'glorification' of 'bestial' appetite is unworthy of godlike man.

This is manifestly garbage. All our principal appetites, from the refinement of whose gratification we derive our most exquisite pleasures and joys, are shared with the beasts. The distinguishing virtue of humans is precisely that we perform rituals and creatively combine the stimuli to our appetites' gratification. Surely it is the man who eats to live or the married couple who dispel sexual appetites in a joyless, one-sided, once-weekly routine, who are performing simply 'bestial' functions?

And then, who is to distinguish between a joyous and sensually pleasurable meal or sexual encounter and, say, fine music or a beautiful painting? All afford sensory pleasure. Through their effects on the senses, they may so elevate the spirit as to afford glimpses of the eternal, but so can massage, drugs, mortification of the flesh or a view of the landscape, but no one would claim for these the status of mere intellectual pleasures, or we would be framing *Times* crosswords and Einstein theorems and hanging them on our walls.

Then there is the argument from 'dignity'. It is claimed that men and women coupling or eating are undignified whilst those in city suits or evening gowns, pontificating or prinking, are dignified.

This raises questions only as to the nature of the entire concept of dignity. For myself, I have never seen a human being so dignified as a greyhound in full pursuit of its prey, or as a horse with its eyes rolling and its flanks darkened and flecked with sweat as it races. Certainly I have never seen human beings approaching such unself-conscious dignity as in nakedness and the unguarded strivings of sex. Then, vulnerable and open as children, they have the beauty of children.

Love then inevitably, and quite properly, enters the equation. I am neither a stranger to love nor sceptical about its virtues. I still hope for – indeed, I believe that I have enjoyed with my swing-partners – the sort of companionable, easy, loyal, unquestioning relationship which provides a secure and contented environment in which creativity and children can thrive.

I just doubt the projection which insists that an enduring relationship must be eternal and eternally sexually exclusive, and make so bold as to assume that sex as necessarily an expression of love – as distinct from the intimacy and companionship bred of shared play and effort – is just a function of social restraints.

So, as nudity is not shameful unless convention demands clothes, so sex is not necessarily and of its nature related to love (as commonly understood) except where pregnancy is likely to be its outcome. Where, in other words, humans are never naked save with their closest intimates, and where sex is presumed to express a willingness to get children, both are, by definition, inalienably expressions of peculiar trust.

Remove such assumptions and sex is itself, and can be enjoyed with all those who stimulate and share the appetite. This is not to say that mutuality, trust and sympathy are not essential to good sex. They certainly are, and the acts of sex, entailing as they do physical intimacy, voluntary vulnerability and intense shared sensation, often engender overwhelming feelings of affection and protectiveness.

I truly believe, however, that I have encountered far more mutuality and sympathy between those who attend orgies in quest of sexual pleasure than in the routine sex enjoyed, often with one partner desirous and the other dutiful, in long-term monogamous relationships, or with both partners desirous to scratch an itch and resorting to mutual exploitation.

7

ELABORATION, ADORNMENT, PROLONGATION, ENRICHMENT ...

'NOPE. CASUAL SEX JUST doesn't do it for me. I've tried,' said Jenny, a 37-year-old mother-of-three, who has had a succession of passionate but disastrous affairs since her divorce. 'I'm a one-man woman. I sometimes wish I wasn't ...'

Jenny is sinuous and lovely. I defy the most resolutely heterosexual female not to glance at her crotch when she walks in tight jeans. She is one of those women whose sexuality sings through denim. We were lovers before she married, enjoyed a drunken and very pleasurable night together after her divorce, but have spent most of our lives as almost-lovers. She had glanced at parts of the manuscript of this book.

Swinging, I told her, bears no relation to casual sex. Casual sex may be equated to the idle snatching-up of snacks or sweets for instant, unthinking gratification. It has no more place in the life of the sexual connoisseur than its equivalent in that of the gastronome.

Like the good cook and host, who works hard at creating conviviality, congeniality, variety and excitement, so the swinger devotes his
or her best efforts to ensuring shared adventure, cultivated pleasures,
a hedonistic merger of imaginations, bodies and intellects.

Eating may serve many purposes. It is, like sex, a simple need, and
there are many who treat sex as the starving treat food. Taste is no
longer important. They want the thing in and for itself, regardless of
where or how they obtain it.

Then, as my doctor friend Johnny had said three years earlier
when I set out on this journey, there are those who eat for reassurance and passing gratification to whom one meal is indistinguishable
in memory from any other. These people also have their counterparts
in the field of sex, regarding it as a necessary if predictable source of
comfort, not as a pleasure to be elaborated upon and pursued, even at
the cost of discomfort and expense.

Gluttons in both are concerned only with repletion, and care little
how it is obtained.

Eating has a high sacramental purpose. So does sex. It would only
be a dangerous fanatic, however, who would restrict his diet to the
host of the Christian Eucharist and consider all other food gross and
unworthy.

And so, in desperation, the critic generally resorts to the patriar-
chal, 'But what about the women involved?' as though he were
asking, 'What of the feelings of the lobster?' when discussing a meal.

'Would you like to see your daughter at an orgy?' one food critic
friend demanded of me when we were on a visit to New Orleans.

This friend had spent the previous evening conventionally at a
casino, a strip-club and a cathouse, I at Colette's swingers' club. The
question was plainly not apposite when asked of the prostitute whom
he had employed.

When I answered, 'Yes, if she were happy,' he professed to be
shocked, and would not speak to me for a full half-hour, and then

only to ask me, in tones of vaguely pitying forbearance though with eagerness barely concealed, what form the previous night's adventures had taken.

Yet when men and women foregather for swinging sex, mutuality and equality are assured as in almost no other sexual activity. The food critic's whore, after all, might have opened her legs to him because she needed drugs or at the behest of a brutal husband or pimp. At best, she had made a reasoned decision that his money justified some discomfort and distaste.

I do not know exactly how my 'oh so respectable' friend had passed his time in the whorehouse, but, even by the dreary actuarial standards of our age, I had certainly enjoyed much better value. He had lost money at a casino and still more in gazing upon women's bodies when he would never have dreamed of similarly paying to look upon a buffet with no prospect of feeding.

He had then, at the further expense of $150, had sex with a woman who, no matter how professional she may have been, was of her nature alien – as well say that you have dined congenially with an unknown waiter – whilst pornographic images flickered on a screen in the corner of the room.

I, on the other hand, had shared jokes with, played with, caressed and been caressed by, some eight or nine attractive women, all fellow members of an international subculture, all bent on their own enjoyment – and, incidentally, had intercourse with four of them – all for an admission fee of $90. Two of those women have since visited me in England and have played both with me and my girlfriend of the time.

As for pornographic images, I had a mind teeming with them, but associated with pleasure and laughter and willing participants rather than paid or coerced performers.

The elaboration, adornment, prolongation and enrichment of the sexual act is, surely, most commonly associated with women. In this regard as in so many others, swinging is a women's world. Men may find basic physiological gratification anywhere. Women demand conditions which make it possible. Swinging affords leisure and luxury, reassurance, conviviality and, perhaps above all, time, without imposing unwanted responsibilities or sacrifice of freedom and autonomy.

Of course there are a few male – and even fewer female – would-be swingers who seems intent upon the urgent gratification of physical appetites, but they are soon shamed by those around them, who will spend many hours in talking and caressing, kissing and tasting, stimulating and sometimes coupling, only to separate and prolong the game. Such people are generally too ashamed to stay long, or to return.

Few players remain in the playrooms for more than an hour or so at a time. There is pleasure to be had in meeting others, in watching others at play, in eating, even in snoozing before returning to the fray.

There is music. There is generally palatable food and drink. The environment is as luxurious as can be contrived. The object is so to heighten pleasure through all the senses that the predictable finality of male orgasm frequently seems irrelevant or downright disappointing.

I have made many good friends through swinging, and yes, sometimes I have had intimate knowledge of their bodies before I have known their names.

What of it? Who ordained the order of such things? No doubt the same moron who laid down the porn film's accelerated *To His Coy Mistress* convention, omitting eyes and brow – sucking breasts, cunnilingus, fellatio, vaginal sex, anal ... I know not a single woman who favours such a simple, dreary narrative thread, relentlessly building to an inevitable and woefully predictable climax.

So, in the non-swinging world, it appears to be accepted that we should meet – preferably by formal introduction – project illusions (for illusion and artifice, whether in male munificence or in female make-up, are at the heart of all seduction, regardless of whether it be sincerely amorous or crassly acquisitive. Seduction is all rhetoric, and all rhetoric lies) and exchange comments about the weather or mutual friends, thus establishing trust and suitability. Thereafter, we may consider thrusting our tongues into and around one another's mouths and faces, and only then can we consider gazing upon or tasting one another's bodies from the neck down.

When we consider that all such rituals are mere substitutes for the no more cursory but probably far more searching canine sniff and lick, but with lies and pretence added on, they seem woefully inadequate as justifications for sexual intercourse and all the implausibly consequent emotional and social commitment: he/she had sex with me and is, therefore 'mine'.

Nor can I look with envy upon those who go through the other ritualistic charades – the shuffling embarrassment and desperate cooing, hooting and yapping of the drinks party, the darkened room in which music reduces conversation to a minimum and a mechanical recorded rhythm replaces and, with luck, prompts, the torpid heartbeat, the lonely charade-parades in winebars where strangers seeking passing reassurance or indiscriminate sexual release encounter those seeking love, and contrive a short- – or, worse, long- – lived compromise.

8

A CAUTIOUS COMMENDATION

IN GIVING A CAUTIOUS, PROVISIONAL commendation to swinging, I do not seek to set it as Rochester does and as Jenny assumed,
against monogamous love, to compare or even to relate them. Any
such comparison would in itself be false, like the misguided debate
between Callicratides and Charicles as to whether a man or a woman
were the appropriate recipient of men's love.

A single monogamous relationship may indeed yield inexpressible
joys to those few able to sustain such a relationship. It would be hard
– and pointless – to dispute whether Monet's repeated exploration of
the same subject in different lights and seasons were more productive
than the more usual serial depiction of multiple subjects.

I am no zealous votary of polygyny or polyandry, prepared like an
arrogant adolescent to scorn the adherents of other systems. Most
swingers, after all, are in long-term monogamous relationships –
which is to say that they do not have 'love' affairs with outsiders.
They simply have sex with other people from time to time as a shared
leisure activity, and consider themselves monogamous.

The only valid comparison, therefore, is between swinging and other extra-marital or socially random sexual transactions, from the casual pick-up to the disregarded but devoted cult, from the laborious and costly invocation of gratitude to the shameful invocation of pity, from the occasional conference hotel room 'romance' to the enduring extra-marital affair. Each of these is essentially solipsistic. Each exploits another emotion or set of emotions in order to win sexual gratification, which may or may not prove emotionally rewarding and may, of course, prove phenomenally destructive.

Swinging is an alternative to such exploits. It is obviously more gregarious, more generally shared between those with social commitments and less susceptible to ambiguous interpretations. It is the pursuit of sexual pleasure, sexual excitement and the liberation of sexually expressed affection in and for themselves.

Swinging has enormous advantages for those temperamentally suited to it. Whether this marks us as a psychological class apart, and whether that class can be deemed (by any save the irredeemably arrogant) emotionally or morally deficient or, indeed, more evolved than others, I certainly would not presume to say. As well argue that those who enjoy dangerous sports, say, or the uxorious, are somehow of their nature 'backward' or preternaturally advanced.

To many of the problems of an age of isolation and confusion as to sexual mores, swinging, for better or for worse, supplies a partial – and often a delightful – solution.

9

A ROMANTIC ENDING?

KATY RETURNED TO THE NORTH and to conventional husband- or partner-seeking, with occasional swinging 'just to keep me sane' and 'to stop me doing anything stupid, like letting some prat take over my life.'

I wanted a new partner, and felt competent at last to seek a woman who would be able to share many other aspects of my life. I was by now confident that I could find her outside the swinging *demi-monde* and that I might yet find someone who, if not committed to swinging full-time, might regard it at least with sympathy and even approval.

Men tend to respond to the word 'swinging' with the usual lascivious nudge and wink and the strange gutshot-bull noise which, in response to mention of communication between genders, indicates the urgent need for bonding with other males. They believe it to be about 'getting their rocks off', but they are also aware of a threat. They must, in their eyes, risk comparison with other males and lose their *de jure* position in the pecking order.

Women, I had discovered, far more readily understand swinging and the moral, spiritual and physical impetuses to it. Although some educated vanilla women in their thirties and forties firmly declared that it wasn't for them (whilst others fetchingly squeaked that they couldn't, really ... they didn't think ...) none told me that it was unthinkable or deplorable.

Initially, this surprised me. On reflection, it is obvious. Women respond to the luxury, the theatricality, the communal nature and the prolonged sensuality of swinging sex. They are already well accustomed to separating their fantasy lives and their obligations, and the formal structuring of swinging, which means that fantasy is not permitted to invade 'real' life, offers rare freedom after a lifetime of repression.

Another friend who had read only parts of this book objected, 'Of course it would be fun, but you're just a cynic. I am a romantic.'

On the other hand, my editor, also an artist, told me, 'My problem is that, if I went swinging, I think I would fall in love with everyone.'

After a moment's hesitation, I told her, 'Yes. I think that is the point. So do I – at least, everyone who is open, vivacious and vulnerable. I suppose that is, ultimately, why I do it.

'And falling in love is such a wonderful thing to do, and far too irresponsible and silly to be influential in real life. It's like a doctor making diagnoses under the influence of acid. But here, I can fall in love and truly love my fellows, give and take in equal measure – and walk away, having learned from them, shared with them and feeling more integrated with my world, whereas in every other form of casual – or, still worse, pseudo-committal – sex, I feel diminished.'

I am, I think, a romantic. I weep at *Casablanca* and the *Enigma Variations*. I yearn for the happy *detentes* of musical comedies. Like Lisa, I even enjoy Georgette Heyer and Mary Stewart.

I believe that most swingers are romantics. They, after all, dress their sexual pleasures up in fantasy and are not content with stagnation and decline, but seek constant renewal and passion.

It is in sharing abandonment that the ultimate pleasure and romance of swinging lies, in the unexpected, touching acts of tenderness, the emergence of the needy, greedy, loving child in the beast, the beast in the man or woman.

For me, who have seen many thousands of people in the exposed extremis of sexual fervour, it is to their hands that my eyes are inevitably drawn. This is not a fetishistic particularity but a distillation of voyeurism – hands trembling, fluttering, flexing, clenching, striking, stroking, soothing, grasping, scratching, probing, seeking – hands, to be thoroughly anthropomorphic, awestruck, wondering, all but autonomous – as at last they are freed to express themselves.

Every one of the successful single male swingers whom I know expresses similar tenderness and wonderment as they describe the continued appeal of swinging when once the obvious, very transitory attractions have lost their novelty. Andy, 34, a soft-spoken divorcee and devoted father, is one of this contingent. He is an East Midlands golf-club professional with a perpetual tan and a notably large cock. We have many couples and female friends in common.

'Yes, it's hands, but toes too, and the things they breathe or shout when they've lost it, and kisses – lots and lots of little kisses – and curling up in your arms and being small and adorable afterwards. So many women look ordinary and self-effacing till you see them like this, naked and playing with their eyes sparkling and their bodies glowing, and then they're so, so beautiful.

'Sometimes I find myself with a woman and I think, "But she's not really my type", but then I find something. It may be in her eyes or in her caresses or in her whimpers or in her taste. There's always something, if she's honest and open and loving, that makes me fall totally in love with her and need to lose myself inside her ...'

There is a distinction to be drawn here between two different concepts of the 'romanticism'. One sort of romantic narrative – the shop girl or mountebank politician variety – requires transfiguration from one state of being to another – from Ugly Duckling to swan, governess to princess, fighting man to beloved memory, doomed, exiled mankind to the New Jerusalem or the vicissitudes of capitalism to the worker state.

Each of these depends upon that most potent and pervasive of lies: that, at the arbitrarily chosen moment of transfiguration, time will stop.

'Happy ever after' usually denotes marriage or sex (or the triumph of the author's ideas), and implies that, now that the hero and heroine have agreed to breed, their natural biological duty to the race is done. They are now, in effect, dead and forever fixed in the oozing resin of romance.

Of course, for real people, marriage or sex (as the reordering of society) is the beginning not of heaven but of heaven knows what problems, including decades of decay. In literature, however, it is a culmination, an apotheosis. All which follows is conveniently concealed from view.

No wonder that so many women, weaned on this lie, feel that there is altogether too much epilogue and too little story.

Death, of course, is an even less questionable and so convenient transfiguration. Even if we no longer posit a heavenly reward or eternal damnation, the dead have moved beyond human dramas and the necessity to question their worth. For them, time has veritably stopped. The date on the gravestone is a full-stop.

It is this sort of romance which swinging very explicitly repudiates.

There is another sort which is braver and more realistic. It acknowledges transience and decay and welcomes both as essential components of beauty and of life itself. It seeks continually to celebrate, enhance and to adorn the raw clay of human existence –

including, for example, genitalia – rather than to despise it and so insist on its transcendence. This is the romance of the artist, the chef and the swinger. It prefers constant renewal and creative muddling to the obsessive pursuit of a dream.

The world would surely be a far happier place had these, rather than their obsessive idealistic brethren, had the running of it.

In the course of my swinging career, then, I have known countless romances – some of a mere few hours' duration, some a few months. Many have become close friendships which find occasional expression in sexual play. Some few have become conventional love affairs in all save our hobby, and might – had it not been for practical factors – have lasted for years.

I consider finding and maintaining such a relationship in future more likely, not less, in consequence of my swinging years. I feel readier (Lord knows, I have had some practice) to essay an enduring love affair than ever before.

When I do so, I will not be freed of the curse of jealousy (deception fractures, and, though the break may knit, it never ceases to hurt when the weather turns cold) but I will at least understand what warrants jealousy and its associated terrors. I will have considerably greater regard for the diversity and exigence of female sexuality. I will be aware that I can and should bring into a relationship what formerly I sought to bring into life by means of my novels – excitement, challenge, adventure, passion, novelty and hugely enhanced sympathy – and that closeness is promoted by all and any shared experience, whilst estrangement is increased by separate fantasy still more than by separate experience.

10

A ROMANTIC BEGINNING

SO HERE, INSTEAD, IS a romantic beginning.

I started a new relationship just three months ago.

There are conventions for such things of course. The shared umbrella or shelter, the accident in the street or the spilled drink, the meeting of eyes across a crowded room, the 'May I have the pleasure ...?'

OK. This one did not quite fit into that mould.

Mandy, a good friend, occasional swing-partner and lover, had come with me to Chameleons. I had been telling her of the supremely comfortable and well-designed sex-swing in the cage-room, so, after a lengthy session with five other couples in the couples' room and a lot of chatting, flirting and oral sex in the bar area, we decided to put it to the test.

As Mandy clasped me around the neck and buttocks, rocked on me and giggled, we struck up a conversation with a couple fucking in the cage behind us. The woman was in her forties, on the burly side but fit, the man greying and very muscular. We chatted about the swing, the club and the cricket. The woman asked if we would like to join them.

I raised an eyebrow at Mandy. She nodded, so we joined them on the cushions. Soon Mandy was on her back, groaning, with the man pounding into her with teeth-jolting force. The woman knelt over her, gasping. Sometimes her mouth was open involuntarily as I fucked her, sometimes voluntarily as she kissed Mandy's face and bobbing breasts.

Suddenly, I felt a tongue lapping between my buttocks. There was a cool finger on either side of my cock. Over my shoulder, I could only see the raised arse of the woman causing me such pleasure. She was callipygian. There were three stars tattooed on her right buttock.

Sex organises itself into movements or chapters with extraordinary spontaneity. Suddenly a change of position or partner is right and inevitable. Mandy was now mumbling and humming (a lot of women seem to hum when eating others. Laura favoured the theme tune from *The Archers*, and certainly the recipients never complained) in the woman's crotch whilst the husband fucked her from behind and the woman and this new girl sucked me. She was in her late twenties, I reckoned, tall, with spiky blonde hair, many tattoos and a pierced clitoris. She gave head with relish and nigh furious enthusiasm.

Now she was sucking the other man. Mandy was still going down on the older woman, but her hand was shepherding and shoving me behind her, so I first caught Christy's eye as I entered another woman and as Christy turned her rump to the burly stranger and he slammed into her, making her breasts flap and the hair spurt from her brow.

She grinned at me – a lovely, riding at speed, free, complicit grin. I liked her. I wanted her.

It was later that Mandy and I met her in the bar and she told us about herself. She was in fact 34. She lived in London. She had been unhappily married and, although a former dancer, had put on over three stones in weight. She had taken a lover who had proved as possessive and proprietorial as her husband. She had persuaded him to give this swinging lark a go.

From the moment that she first visited Swingers' Junction in Hampshire, she said, she had felt at ease and at home. The boyfriend had felt threatened by it and had left. She had been swinging as a single female for the past six months. She was now back to 8st 4lbs. She had come here tonight with – a mistake.

She had responded to an advertisement on Local Swingers. A single male called Martin had invited her to spend the weekend with him. She had been impressed by his literacy, his apparent sensitivity and wit and, she admitted, his Jaguar.

She had arrived this afternoon in Droitwich, however, to find that he was an ageing student living with several others at a cottage on his father's land, that the Jag was his father's and that one of his female housemates had written his profile and his email for him. Worse, Martin was 'a wanker who has no idea what this is all about. Seems to think it's a glorified freebie lapdance.'

'If I could write songs, I'd write one called *I Went to Bed with a Headache and Woke up with a Jerk*,' she giggled. 'Story of my life.'

Mandy liked this a lot. 'So what have you done with him?' she asked.

'Oh, I tried to introduce him to some people. He just goggled and leered. I think he's in the jacuzzi with his tongue hanging in the water. I came to find you guys instead.'

It turned out that she had heard about me from some couples with whom I had played. She had been intrigued. She had watched me and, apparently, the faces of the five women (she, like several women whom I know, loves to watch other girls' faces as they are fucked, especially by her man) in the couples' room as we had played. She had decided that she wanted to get to know me. 'So,' she said as she downed her drink. 'Shall we go and play?'

So the three of us went and played in the red room for a couple of hours, and Christy's fingers clung and caressed and sometimes she was wild and slavering and gave off great bellows as she came, and sometimes her kisses were small and needy and passionate, and she loved my face and all the neglected parts of the body. We played there with three other couples, but all the time she retained eye contact with me and returned into my arms.

Mandy could see what was happening. She suggested that Christy escape her partner and accompany us back to our hotel room. We all spent that night together. Mandy had to leave at ten in the morning to take her son to a rugby match, so she kissed us and left us with instructions to look after one another. We made love, then, had brunch at a roadside bistro and returned to Chameleons for a leisurely afternoon.

Christy has been with me almost every weekend since then, and we have walked the dog and gone surfing and gone out to dinner and stayed with friends, and argued and made up and enjoyed trips to Paris and Prague like all lovers.

Oh, and we have fucked quite a lot of people along the way.

As with any vanilla relationship, by the time that this is read, we may of course no longer be a team. Long-range relationships are never easy to maintain. We may have resolved to move closer to one another. We will still – and always, I suspect – be friends. All my former lovers with whom I have played are still close. We call one another late at night, compare notes, discuss relationships and work. We have shared too much, and are not subject to the horrors of sexual jealousy and resentment which make a rift – and even hatred – so essential in those relationships whose intimacy is defined by exclusive sex.

I ventured into this world more or less *faute de mieux*, motivated by curiosity and a desire for safe play amidst congenial companions. After three years, I cannot conceive of a better, kinder, warmer, happier, more robust, more libertarian world than that which I found just below the crackling lacquer surface of our own society.

My probationary period is over. I can now consider a more exacting relationship with the blessing of my Minnesota Method counsellors. I am still sober, and have found a means to ecstasy far more efficacious and less injurious than most. I have learned a huge amount – not academically, but intuitively – about my fellows and their healthy but repressed longings.

Above all (and, as one with prodigious appetites reared a Catholic, I can say this of few other such periods in my life) I can look back on three years' swinging with a clear conscience. I have given, and shared in, an enormous amount of carefree, childlike, hedonistic fun without doing harm.

I, like countless romantics before me, have travelled the world in search of 'innocence'. I found it just down the road, amidst the groans, gasps, grunts and giggles of an orgy.

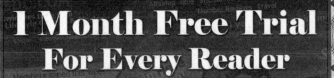